Finding Time To Care For Me

A Nurse's Guide to Self-Care

MIA REDRICK

LORNA IMPERIAL

Finding Definitions, LLC
P. O. Box 68045
Baltimore, MD 21215

Library of Congress Cataloging-in-Publication Data
Finding Time to Care for Me: A Nurse's Guide to Self-Care
ISBN 9780979627323 (tradepaper)
  • Self-Help I. Redrick, Mia II. Imperial, Lorna
  • Nursing

Printed in the United States of America
Printed in the United States by Lightning Source Inc.

For information about special discounts for bulk purchases, please contact
Finding Definitions Sales at 1-866-226-2607 or info@findingdefinitions.com.

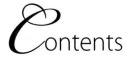

Contents

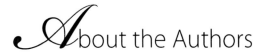bout the Authors

Mia Redrick

Mia and her husband of 13 years reside in Maryland with their three children. Mia is an author, radio host, motivational speaker and self-care strategist. She speaks throughout the country on topics of concern to caregivers and nurturers.

Lorna Imperial

Lorna Imperial, RN MSN PhD MCC CIMP, is a highly educated, well respected and experienced nurse, entrepreneur, and educator. Her background encompasses a wide cross section of nursing administration, medical / surgical, psychiatric, critical care, community health, and other specialties. Lorna has successfully blended strong educational ethics with real-world wisdom and experience.

Lorna has 2 daughters. Lorna is married to a physician and lives in Maryland.

*B*lending of Talents and Skills

Finding Time for Me: The Nurses Guide to Self-Care is a book that shows you how to make time in your busy life to acknowledge and nurture your individual needs while maintaining your daily schedule. This book shows you how reclaiming your individuality also makes you a better caregiver.

The writers, Mia Redrick and Lorna Imperial, have successfully blended their collective talents and expertise to produce a step-by-step approach that is both successful, and easily integrated into your daily life as a health care provider.

Mia Redrick, a successful self-care coach, radio host and motivational speaker shares her turn-key self-care system that empowers healthcare professionals to practice better self-care.

Lorna Imperial's vast expertise as an RN and outstanding International Meeting Planner specializing in "self-care cruises", has allowed this team to marry both experience and expertise to address the needs of those that care for others.

Together Mia and Lorna provide the answers for nurses to find time, grow personally, self-connect and assign meaning to their lives. Practical and inspirational, "Time for me" will teach you powerful strategies to practice daily self-care essential steps to refueling the nurturer.

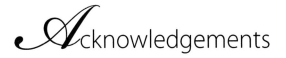

Acknowledgements

From Mia

Taking the steps to pursue your dreams is a daily decision. The support, encouragement and love of others often allow our dreams to take flight. I am very fortunate to have great wingmen and wing-women. They are:

Patrick (my hubby): Thank you for understanding my vision. I appreciate the commitments that you have made to help me make my dreams possible. I am blessed to have your support and love. Big hugs and kisses, and loads of love!

Patrick, Alexandra and Matthew: You are the best children ever! I appreciate all of your advice, support, and understanding that writing a book takes commitment. I love you all.

Mom and Dad: Mom, thank you for teaching me the importance of self-care from the beginning of my early days as a mom. Dad, I appreciate your example that everything is possible. I love you both.

James, Michelle and Taylor and Ashley: James you are the funniest brother around. You always make me smile. Michelle, I am blessed to have you as my sister-in-law. Taylor and Ashley, you are the best nieces in the world.

Coach T.: You are the best coach in the Universe. You have

always made requests of me that have allowed me to own my best and reach for more. Love Ya.

Doc. Delia and Melva: You are the best running buddies a girl could ask for. You are terrific doctors. I am glad that the world finally knows. I appreciate your expertise, wisdom and support.

Miameesha: Thank for all your support and hard work. You are the best.

Michelle C.: Your support always touches me and reminds me of the benefit of great friendships.

Wayne and Kenneth Clapp: Thank you for the beautiful photos for this book.

Linda at Wordpros, Woody and Anne Henslee: You are the best editors in the world. Thank you for excelling in the English language.

Andrea B: Everyone needs an honest friend. You are mine.

Winston you are an amazing mentor. Thank you for everything.

Ty Howard: Thank you for setting the pace my friend.

Glenn Garnes you are such a go-giver.

Patsy Anderson: You example of business ownership is an incredible gift. Thank you for sharing it with me.

Austin Duncan: Quiet Brilliance.

The Power Team: I am blessed to mastermind with you all.

Last but not least, my clients. Thank you all for validating that personal coaching is essential to a person's growth and development. I respect all of you and have learned from your willingness to be your personal best.

> Remember to always. . .
> Live Fully.
> Mia

From Lorna

I want to say thank you to everyone for all the support you have given, and the friendships I have established along the way.

Special thanks to the following special people in my life:

Ed: "The Spotlight of my Life".

Christine & Guinevieve: For teaching me to take care of myself first based on the concept of "Mom-Me & Foremost".

To my Mom-Mely: I learned so much from you. You proved my success theory. I am successful. Thank you.

Patsy A: For all the connections.

Mary Ann: For all the care and budgetary support.

Vickie R.: For operational support and great ideas.

Bob B.: Media & exposure for our group.

Deanna L.: For technology support and educational guidance.

Austin D.: Your simple tech solutions and brilliant ideas.

Jun P. & Emilie D.: For your constant pursuit of good projects towards humanity.

Emma D.: For your encouragement to be active on medical missions.

To all the nurses whom I have worked with over the years, I'd like to say that my experience with each of you played an important role in sculpting my successful nursing career.

Bless you all.
Lorna

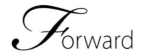orward

As nurses and health care professionals our world runs on high-octane fuel. Many times it seems as if we live a life of demands, not a life devoted to self-actualization. We keep asking the question, "Where is the time going?" noticing how quickly our lives are moving. At times we feel like spectators playing important roles in the lives of others when in fact we should be the leading character.

As a person moves into the role of caregiver, they go through change, expansion, fear, growth, and even shrinkage. Caregivers become focused on the care of others such that they often lose touch of wants, desires, and personal needs. Everything we do; reading, listening, reacting – it's all tied to caring for someone else in an indirect way.

Society has little to say as a culture about how nurses care for nurses. It's taken for granted that because this is our chosen career path that we willingly give up self. We come to accept this definition as universal truth. We ignore the needs, wants, desires, and individual tenets that make us unique as a person settling for membership into a growing subset of falsehoods.

Nurses' days are long filled with many complex and some-times heart wrenching tasks. We feel for others and want to make a difference in their lives. It hurts us when we must perform procedures that we know cause our patient's pain – yet it's for their own well being and in their best interest. Those thoughts of empathy tend to flash-back in our minds when we least expect them and if affects our lives in ways not realized. We go home to our families without leaving the role of caregiver on the unit. We become defined by what we do, not who we are.

That is about to change. You are about to reclaim yourself as an individual defined as a unique person who happens to be a nurse.

One of the best ways for nurses to get support, insight, inspiration, advice and answers is through the coaching process. Coaching provides you with the opportunity to explore your own feelings about life and to help you get back your sense of humor in dealing with day-to-day issues. Coaching is like having your own personal support system.

Through the coaching approach in this book, you will learn to take better care of yourself and create strategies to create inner peace and calm, to recharge and refresh yourself. You will feel more power, greater self-confidence and will be happier in your role of being a nurse. This book focuses on the complete you, not just the nurse. When you invest in time for "Me", your whole world profits.

Sincerely,
Lorna Imperial

*H*ow to use
Finding Time to Care for Me:
A Nurse's Guide to Self-Care

Finding Time for Care for Me: A Nurse's Guide to Self-Care was originally created as a resource for anyone who defines herself as a mom. It quickly became apparent that nurses share the same set of responsibilities – especially towards self. Health care professionals give so much to others that they quickly lose sight of what is important in their individual lives.

To make the most of reading this book I encourage you to answer the questions honestly, quietly and reflectively. The purpose of the assignments is to get you to think about your life and to aid you in altering the habits, routines, relationships, along with the processes and infrastructure that prevent you from living the life about which you dream. It's not about redefining your role in life, but about recapturing your unique individuality.

This book was written with an understanding of the busyness of a health care professional's life. As nurses and health care professionals, it is even more important that you allow yourself to not only be happy, but fulfilled. In giving to yourself, you give to others. This book is designed as a simple, but powerful resource to help move you toward actions that will assist you in recreating and renegotiating a life that is rich, fulfilling and meaningful.

Before beginning any chapter, I recommend that you close your eyes and empty your thoughts. Let go of the stress and schedule for the day. Take a deep breath and breathe in and out slowly to relax your body. Take a minimum of 15 minutes each day to read this book and complete the assignments and practices. Remember to focus only on you while reading this book.

At the end of each chapter, there is an affirmation for you to sign and date, *"I took an action for me today and it felt great!"* The goal is to help you build the muscle of doing something to improve your life every day by taking small steps. Be sure to journal after reading each chapter to record your thoughts.

Throughout the chapters there are various assignments and practices. Although you might want to skip ahead to the next chapter, if this is your first time reading this book, it is recommended that you completely finish one chapter before moving to the next. All of the chapters are building blocks to help you redevelop patterns that will help you move forward easily.

Connect to a community for accountability

✓ Join with your local nurses group. Even better, form a group with other nurses that share your unique interests and goals.

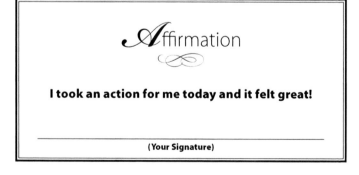

*A*ffirmation

I took an action for me today and it felt great!

_____
(Your Signature)

✓ Start a nurses group dedicated to building a support system for one another. No one understands nurses like other nurses.

✓ Partner with your friends, coworkers, or family members who care about your well-being. Your circle of potential friends includes people from all walks of life. This diversity enhances your life by allowing you to see things from another's viewpoint and mindset.

Share your success with us at www.findingdefinitions.com/caregivers.html

I welcome the opportunity to help you get started on this exciting journey towards self-definition. I am thrilled for you, and I will be there with you every step of the way.

Live Fully,
Mia

$\mathcal{H}$ow to use Finding Time to Care for Me, Nuture-Me Journal Sections

---

Congratulations on your purchase of *Finding Time to Care for Me: The Nurses Guide to Self-Care,* and on making the decision to commit to yourself. This journal section serves as a guide to help you enhance the current blueprint for your life. As nurses, we become so busy taking care of our families and patients that we forget to listen to our own voice. This journal will help you find your voice and discover who you are again.

Journaling daily will help you keep a written record of your life. As nurses, we become so busy with the demands of work, family, and home that we forget to consider how we feel as a unique individual. The journaling component was created specifically for you to write about your life as an individual who just happens to be a nurse. Each day, take fifteen minutes to record how you feel about your life. Write about your thoughts and feelings about yourself, your day, or anything that you wish. If you get stuck, I have created a list of questions at the end of each chapter for you to consider when journaling. Choose one or two questions from my list to help you get started. I encourage you to add your own questions to this list that reflects your unique situation.

The goal is for you to begin to hear from yourself again. I want you to have a written record of the things that you want to keep in your life and the things that you want change. Taking the time everyday to hear your inner desires is the best way to *Live Fully.*

Suggested Journal Questions:

1. What do I want for my life? Who am I? What do I like about my life? What do I want to change? What is working? What is not?

2. How do I feel? What in my life brings me the greatest joy? What brings me the least enjoyment? What do I do for pleasure? How do I relax?

3. When was the last time I reflected on me? How do I renew and rejuvenate myself? When was the last time I was still?

4. Do I feel powerful or powerless? Why? What are my boundaries? Do I exercise choice in my life? Do I trust myself?

5. Why do I love me? What am I grateful for? What are my priorities? What can I celebrate about me? Do I show myself love? How? When?

6. What is your life telling me? What do you need to get rid of?

7. What opportunities are around you? What is your dream? What is your purpose?

8. When was the last time I was alone? How much rest do I need? When was the last time I cried? When was the last time I laughed?

9. What makes me smile? Am I dancing to the music of life or is it just background music?

10. Do I enjoy my friendships? What kind of friend am I? When was the last time you helped someone in need without expecting anything in return?

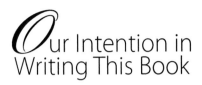

Our Intention in Writing This Book

Our intention in writing this book is to create both a dialogue and a supportive community among individuals as nurses that address the realities of a working professional as they relate to self-definition. Our goal is to provide you with strategies and solutions that will set you on a path to find meaningful ways to incorporate yourself into your life as a person who is not solely defined by your chosen trade.

Considering the steps that you must take is essential for any person who wants more out of life—specifically as you share with others in one of the most demanding fields imaginable. We all want the same —things: happy families, a secure financial life, and friends and family members that care for us, we also want to be happy ourselves.

We have found that the personal happiness of an individual directly contributes to a happy family.

If you were asked to write your personal entry in the Webster's Dictionary today of your definition of nurse and the definition of me, what would you say? Perhaps your definitions might say something like this:

> **Nurse**: (nurse)
> *Noun*
> *Definition:* A person educated and trained to care for
> the sick or disabled; one that serves as a nurturing
> or fostering influence in the lives of others.

Me: (me)
Pronoun
Definition: A person who loves, nurtures, fosters, protects, teaches

Your turn! Write your definition of "Nurse" and then your definition of "Me."

Nurse (nurse)
Noun
Definition:

Me (me)
Pronoun
Definition:

What are your observations about your definitions? Are you surprised by the level of challenge that this simple exercise caused you?

We created this program to help nurses expand their limited definition of themselves as individuals. As health care professionals, it is even more important you achieve self-actualization. Our goal is to challenge nurses to live fully, be healthy, dream big and personally grow in their own lives. While there is no one-size-fits-all strategy for self care, we propose throughout this book the essential guidelines for placing yourself at the top of the list.

We decided to write this book because we have read countless books on helping people find balance. The truth of the matter is that balance is not something we find; it is something we create.

Live Fully,
Mia and Lorna

What is Finding Definitions?

Finding Time to Care for Me: The Nurse's Guide to Self-Care was created to teach others that self-care is not negotiable, but necessary to be the best person possible. As a personal coach strategist, I ask my clients the tough questions to unlock their answers for a happier life. Through a series of my questions, you will better be able to identify who you are and what you want for your life.

Finding Definitions helps health care professionals:

Find Time ....To Self Accomplish

Find Balance .... To Enjoy Each Day

Find Meaning.................................... To Listen to Your Voice

Find Connection .... To Establish Supportive Networks

Find You.. To Discover Who You Are

Find Gratitude ....To Acknowledge
What Makes You Happy

This is not an ordinary book. *This book* is specifically designed for nurses to encourage them to be honest about their lives. I want you to Reflect, Release, Renew and Resolve. It is my hope that this book and the journaling will aid you in creating the life you want.

Use it daily to challenge yourself with the tough questions about the quality of your life. Visit my website at www.findingdefinitions.com/caregivers.html for additional resources on assigning meaning to your life as a person and a health care professional.

Thank you in advance for making you a priority.

Live Fully,
Mia

Chapter 1
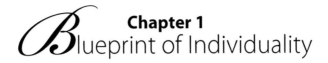
Blueprint of Individuality

Being an individual changes everything!

When we become nurses, it changes our routines, patterns, the way we love and feel love. Never before did we know it was possible to love others the way we do now. As we evolve as health care professionals, we find it more difficult and less important to continue to do for ourselves as we did before.

It was never our intention to lose ourselves; it just happened as part of this new set of expectations, obligations and the abyss of the unknown. We would have been ahead of the curve had we really understood the impact of the profession on our lives and why it was stressed in nursing school that we must take care of ourselves first in order to be of service to others.

In fact, working in nursing is like being thrown a curveball. Just when you think you know what you are doing, you find yourself somewhere else and learning something new. There are times you go to work, clock in, and start your routine on your usual floor. One of the first things you do is sign in on the nursing sign in sheet. Then you see the inevitable: You're assigned to float to a floor you've never been on, with patients you've never seen, in a specialty you've never worked and with other nurses that you don't know. Your heart beats – for a very brief moment you think of feigning sick. Dread builds. You don't even know where the soiled utility room is – much less where to the crash cart if you need it.

You smile at your coworkers and head to the elevator. You just intercepted that curveball. What you do with it is up to you.

My mother said to me soon after my son was born that being a mother is *what you do* not *who you are*. I remember thinking at the time that this was insane. **Being a mother is who I am now.** I am a mother. I have waited all my life for this moment and now I am a mother. But my own mother was absolutely right. Being a parent is playing a role, a role that many people developed from their earliest experiences. That same analogy can be used in nursing.

What made you want to become a nurse? Is being a nurse what you thought it would be? What are the curveballs you have been thrown? Is being a nurse what you do, or does it define you as an individual?

What adjectives do you use to describe a nurse?

Being a mom describes just one aspect of who I am as a person. What my mom wanted me to understand from the beginning is that being a good mom had much to do with my ability to be good to myself. And there are many ways to be good to you too.

As caregivers, we learn early in our lives that we have an inherent need to help and nurture others. Nurses play the same role at work. Many times when I am conducting a workshop, I ask the participants to look for similarities between themselves and their past influences. Many of us pick up behaviors and attitudes from our past without thinking about it. I call this our blueprint.

What is your *Nurture-Me* script?

Have you placed limitations on what you can achieve? Are

you unsure how you have created the life you have gotten? Let's explore your nurture-Me script. In order to accurately assess your current behaviors, complete the following exercise while being completely honest. Use your journal to detail your responses.

Nurture "Me" Assessment

Consider the following:

1. Growing up, I best remember the atmosphere at home as (i.e. controlling, permissive, detached, strained, etc...).

2. I can best describe my individual style as (i.e. controlling, permissive, detached, easy-going, etc...).

3. How has your past influenced your present? Do you see any similarities or striking differences based on your childhood experiences?

4. Growing up, I (always, occasionally, never) found time for myself and my own interests. -

5. Or...My time was always structured because...

6. As an adult individual, I (always, occasionally, never) find time for myself. When I do, I...Or...I never find time because (I work too much overtime, I'm just too tired...)

7. Do you see any similarities or differences based on your childhood experiences?

8. MY favorite part of being with my family was...

9. How did this affect your life?

10. I did not enjoy some parts of my life growing up because…

11. How has this influenced you as an adult?

12. Do you do the same, total opposite, or somewhere in between?

13. What questions would you like to add about your Nurture-"Me" script?

A nurturing script many times causes us to continue to do the same things we did when we were growing up. Many people begin by using their past experiences as a template and as the basis for their own family and personal life in adult-hood. Do you?

The purpose of raising these issues is to make you conscious of why you "feel the way that you do. One of the best ways to understand your life is by making powerful observations and by asking yourself the right questions about your habits, thoughts and feelings. Throughout this book I will help you make those observations and ask you the right questions to unlock the answers inside of you.

Marisa's mom, Kelly, worked part-time and was always home for the children by the time they got out of school. She was a happy person but always made sure that professional and personal commitments did not interfere with her time with the children. She volunteered at church a couple of times a week and kept her schedule clear for the children's commitments.

Marisa, now a nurse herself, followed the same routine. She liked her life but had no idea why she operated the way she did. She came to me because she wanted to start a business and could not see how it was possible.

Lorna says: Can you see how our past experience influences our present? Stop and list three influences that you carry into adulthood from your past.

The Silent War

There is a silent war that threatens the uncultivated self. This silent war is a lack of self-care and it operates like one big muscle. If we fail to exercise, it becomes flabby and out of shape. This the lack of self-care surfaces slowly and quietly. We can no longer identify what we like to read or movies we enjoy seeing. Sometimes we are too busy to add our own needs to the list. We are no longer multi-tasking professionals; we are mega-tasking in machine-like fashion. The stress of caring for others during our work day tends to come home with us as well.

This silent war defeats us when we stop knowing ourselves. For most it is a gradual process of developing habits and thoughts which make us feel selfish for wanting to have hobbies, quality friendships, and romantic dates with our significant other…much less professional careers. Logic dictates that it is impossible to do all of these things and still please everyone around us.

The silent war often goes on for years until one day we realize that we have become unfamiliar with the person we once were. We are unable to identify the simple things; such as our favorite restaurants, outfits that look best on our bodies outside of scrubs, music we love, movies we want to see, or places we love to visit. What would you add to this list?

I have spoken with many nurses regarding this process of

silently fading away. The irony for many is while our lives are fading, others in our lives are thriving. Somehow as nursing professionals we manage to coordinate the care of our patients, answering call lights, pass meds, deliver meal trays, deal with physicians – and then do charting and paperwork. We do all of this and keep up with the state mandated continuing education credits, get to work early to get report, stay late to finish charting – and this does not include the inevitable extended shift. Is it any wonder that we fail to create time for ourselves? We have an internal war that says *"Not now." "There isn't enough time or resources." "Just wait until...my days off... off-peak season hits...my vacation,"* or whatever your reason is for putting yourself on hold. Is this you? Are you making these false assumptions?

Stop and think:

If you were the patient, what would your wellness nursing diagnosis be?

If you had a patient in your charge who felt as if they had lost a sense of self, how would you council them?

Many times your patients are not able to identify the cause of their ailments. Are you able to identify the cause of yours? Have you become so used to feeling empty and tired that it has become part of your persona?

The Assumptions of Nursing

FALSE ASSUMPTIONS	TRUE ASSUMPTIONS
I am Super-Nurse and can handle anything thrown at me. Nursing diagnosis: Potential for personal breakdown due to overwork, juggling responsibility, and health problems related to chronic stress.	In this profession, it's amazing how you can literally save someone's life and get no credit for it, but if you accidentally forget to unclamp your secondary tubing for your IV antibiotic, you will hear about it for weeks.
I am a nurse because I am a kind, compassionate person who has a great desire to help people. Nursing diagnosis: Potential for burnout due to taking on too many responsibilities.	Many nurses have that kindness and compassion. But take years of being stepped on by patients, families, co-workers, and administration and those feelings will be replaced by bitterness to a degree. It's only natural.
I don't mind going in to work a 12-hour shift, and then have the nurse manager extend it to a 16-hour shift – three times a week – with no advance notice. Nursing diagnosis: Potential for animosity to build placing a strain on existing relationships with self and others. Potential for physical and mental exhaustion related to overwork.	It only takes a few rude, manipulative, drug-seeking patients (you know, the ones rating their pain at a 10/10 asking for 3mg of IV Dilaudid-all while laughing on the phone and eating a bag of chili-cheese Fritos) to stress you out. Combine this with the shortage of nurses and the daily interaction with patients and it's no wonder relationships are strained.

I leave the unit as soon as I can, and get into my car to drive home, I feel like I've been released from prison. But that's alright, I can deal with it. The paycheck is worth it. Nursing diagnosis: Potential for medical and mental stress related anomalies caused from lack of self-care.	Self-care is a mindset that establishes your life with you at the top of the list. Understand that if you take care of you, you will be better able to care for others. Your self-image will improve, your anxiety level will decrease, and you will feel happier about yourself as an individual and as a nurse.
I'm torn between feeling like I should be earning a certain amount, because I shouldn't waste the degree, or doing something I'd really consider fun, but living on a low income. Nursing diagnosis: Possible misconceptions which may lead to exacerbation of depression, stress, anxiety, and feelings of negative self-worth. Potential for strained relationships, loss of enjoyment of life, and long-term health problems.	While earning a living at nursing, you can also apply your skills to a passion that you love. If you love to paint but haven't sold any paintings, try networking with other nurses. You are responsible for your own happiness as an individual.

Lorna Says: Write one nursing diagnosis for you:	As a nurse, write your action plan here:
Problem:	
Potential for:	
Related to:	
Possible Consequences:	

_____

_____

_____

_____

_____

_____

_____

_____

_____

_____

_____

_____

_____

_____

_____

_____

_____

_____

_____

_____

_____

_____

_____

_____

_____

_____

_____

_____

_____

_____
_____
_____
_____
_____
_____
_____
_____
_____
_____
_____
_____
_____
_____
_____
_____
_____
_____
_____
_____
_____
_____
_____
_____
_____
_____
_____
_____

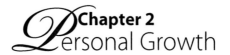

Chapter 2
Personal Growth

Think of yourself as your favorite piece of jewelry. What does your favorite piece of jewelry look like when it is dirty? Does it shine or reflect light? The same is true with our lives when we fail to polish, buff or enhance ourselves by personally growing. We stop shining, singing, and reflecting the light that is inside of us. That may mean we are not as happy or fulfilled as we can be.

As individuals who make it our profession to give to others in countless and selfless ways, we lose a sense of true self. As a result, we stop growing; we stop knowing ourselves. Remember when you used to accomplish something different for yourself every day? Remember how you felt? When we stop doing the little things for ourselves that we once did, like pursuing hobbies, making friends outside of our profession and looking our best when we are not in scrubs, we stop knowing how to accomplish those things.

Personal growth is cultivating yourself in ways that leave you changed for the better. When we take the time to look our best, we change the way we see ourselves and we change how others see us. When we take the time to create meaningful adult relationships, we are supported, validated, and provided with a network of resources for ourselves.

What is Personal Growth for Nurses?

Personal growth is recognizing that we have the capacity

to be more of who we already are. We are sympathetically aware that each of us has the ability to grow, enhance and evolve as a person. When we grow, we are able to enrich those around us as well as ourselves. We are able to work toward our goal of personal excellence and expand our gifts, talents and potential.

As health care professionals, many times we feel stifled by our busy schedules or unscheduled interruptions at work—like stat physicians orders, a patient who codes unexpectedly, or administrative politics work. One thing you are always guaranteed as a nurse; your days may not always go according to plan. To ensure your success you have to have a mindset that is specific about what you are trying to accomplish—for you—every day—all day.

As nurses, we sometimes stop growing personally because of life's distractions. Finding ways to balance the noise of work, home commitments, family and self seems daunting. Most times the transitions or unscheduled interruptions get us off track and result in our creating habits that are not helpful. Though it might be challenging to partially self-accomplish only during our off hours, this needs to become a true mindset so that we can follow through on the little things that add up.

The Benefits of Personal Growth

✓ **To be happy with your life.** Happy people make happy families.

✓ **To reclaim the beautiful art of cultivating the self. Nurses!** Reclaim YOU!

✓ **Recognizing that we can always evolve.** Evolution is change in progress!

✓ **To increase our ability to have meaningful relationships with others.** Make connections that improve your life.

✓ **To provide ourselves with creative outlets that allows us to share ourselves with the world.** Growing is not about checking off a list of things to do, but instead doing something as an expression of joy or self-worth.

✓ **Growing means we are moving to enhance our life not growing to reach a specific destination.** Make time to enjoy the journey.

✓ **Growing means showing yourself love.** You deserve love, don't you? Don't forget the importance of treating yourself.

What is Your Life's Reflection?

The following assessment was created to help you learn about your life. Answer these questions honestly with the intention of getting some understanding about areas that are ripe for growth. Use your journal to detail your responses.

Nurture "Me" Assessment

Consider the following:

Financial

1. What would you like to create financially?
2. What are your financial goals? Do you ever think about creating wealth?
3. What resources do you currently utilize to keep a record of your finances?

4. Do you have an understanding of your work and household expenses?
5. Do you know how to locate your financial information and resources easily?
6. Do you pay your expenses on time?
7. Do you live a life that you can afford?
8. What other questions would you like to ask yourself about your finances?

Work/Career
1. Are you happy in your career as a nurse?
2. What could make your work life better?
3. What could you do right now to change your work situation?
4. Name three things you are merely tolerating in your work.
5. What steps do you need to take to eliminate these from your life immediately?
6. Does your work allow you to express your true talent or is it just a decent paycheck?
7. Do you often feel physically and mentally exhausted at the end of your work day? Why?
8. What elements are missing from your work life?

Legacy
1. Are you living the life you always envisioned?
2. What shifts would you like to make to attain your dream life?
3. How do you want to be remembered as a nurse...a wife...a husband...an individual?

Hobbies
1. What are your hobbies outside of the medical field?
2. When was the last time you spent time on these hobbies?
3. How did you feel while doing this activity?
4. Why don't you have hobbies?
5. Do you feel guilty when having personal fun?

Health
1. When did you last visit your doctor?
2. Why haven't you gone to the doctor? (Being a nurse is beside the point.)
3. Are you healthy?
4. Do you exercise outside of walking the hospital floors? How often? Why not?
5. What does your ideal health look like for you?
6. What resources do you have at your disposal to exercise?
7. What type of exercise do you like?
8. What is an easy way for you to exercise?

Relational
1. Write down your five most important relationships.
2. Describe the type of influence these relationships have on you (e.g., supportive, demanding, needy).
3. Do you feel loved?
4. Who understands you best?
5. Do you want to establish meaningful relationships?
6. Are your only friends other nurses? If so, why?
7. Do you have relationships that inspire you?
8. Who is you confidante?

Personal
1. What about your life makes you happy?
2. How do you feel when you are happy?
3. Who are you? (How do you describe yourself to others?)
4. What are you most grateful for in your life?
5. How does this make you feel?
6. What makes you proud in your life?
7. What about this makes you feel good?
8. What do you like about yourself?

Answering the questions in this simple assessment gives you some perspective on areas with potential for personal growth. These questions are meant to be guidelines and not a complete list. What other questions do you need to ask yourself about these areas of your life? What do you really want?

The purpose of this assignment is to get you used to seeing your life completely instead of in fragments. I believe that personal growth should be reflected in various areas of our lives.

The areas of personal growth are referred to as the **Wheel of Our Lives.** There are eight areas of our lives that require personal growth or attention to live a balanced life. The areas are as follows:

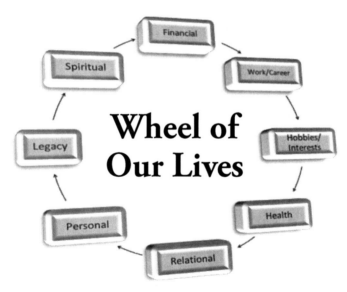

Areas of Balanced Life

Financial	Enhancing the economic security and increasing awareness of the family's financial picture.
Productive Work/Career/ Outlet	Establishing opportunities which allow you to express yourself productively either in or outside of the home. This includes being in touch with yourself so that you can say a resounding "No!" when you have to.
Hobbies/ Recreational	Creating meaningful channels to express your passion(s) allowing you to stay connected to your interests.
Health	Maintaining good physical health by utilizing exercise to energize, relieve stress and reduce anxiety.
Relational	Establishing supportive networks that validate you and provide resources for living life to its fullest.
Personal	Creating opportunities to feel, express and enjoy no matter where you are.
Contribution/ Legacy	Creating a life that has meaning and value which allows you to support your family but leaves evidence of living fully while giving of yourself in your chosen profession.
Spiritual	Creating a means to refuel spiritually by being reflective, prayerful, or engaging in a fellowship of worship.

As we understand ourselves as individuals, we know we are not single-faceted, but conversely, we are multidimensional.

When we consider our areas of personal growth, we must also consider the various stages of growth. I believe that to be a whole person you must accomplish several of these developmental areas at the same time. Yes, it is possible to take care of your physical health and grow intellectually while having friendships that you honor. Many times we pick from a small list for ourselves, believing that our world needs to be small in order to manage the demands of home and career.

Understanding this, I created a definition for the stages of personal growth for nurses. They are the following: **Stagnant, Motion, Acceleration.**

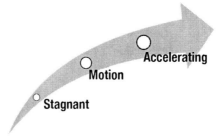

You may look at the Nurture-"Me" Wheel and determine that you are only accomplishing progress in a few of these areas, or you may notice that you have consistently maintained your relationship with friends and family, but at the expense of your health. Still, there are several other areas that await you. Take your time, but make the decision to cultivate growth in each of these eight areas.

The first stage of personal growth is STAGNANT

Stagnant means that any growing that happens is void of real change. When you are stagnant in your personal growth, you are continuing to do, wear, look, and feel the same every day. This stage is easy because life is comfortable and familiar.

People who are stagnant may do any of the following:
- Wear the same clothes multiple times of the week
- Fail to fix their hair in the morning
- Not exercise
- Eat unhealthy foods
- Feel sadness but not know why
- Lack energy
- Lack emotion
- Feel irritable

The reason we feel this way is because each day presents the same mundane routine. We may feel just like a hamster on a wheel. We may feel our lives are moving, but going nowhere. Admittedly, this is a hard stage to change, especially for the health care professional.

The strategies necessary to change this stage are:

1. **Identify possible areas of growth.** Circle the areas on the Personal Growth Wheel where you would like to improve in your life.
   > Financial
   > Work/Career
   > Hobbies/Recreational
   > Health
   > Relational
   > Personal
   > Legacy
   > Spiritual

2. **Ask yourself the following questions:**
   (a) What shifts can I make in this ___ of my life?

    (b) What is missing in this area of my life?

    (c) What would I like to see in this area?

    (d) What ability do I have right now to create this change?

3. Map your behavior as you change:

    (a) Practice makes perfect. Start slowly and begin with one area.

    (b) Allow for transition. Initially you will feel awkward working on this area of your life, because it is unfamiliar. Be patient with yourself. Give yourself time to feel positive about this new change.

    (c) Reward yourself and feel good about making strides. Examples of rewards include the following: get a pedicure/manicure, plan a date with your favorite book in the park, take a walk in a scenic location, or give yourself a facial. Now what reward will you choose?

    (d) Repeat this step until it becomes a habit.

Mastering it is the goal.

4. Define your values. Do you know what you value? Do you value rest and clarity of thought? Do you value creativity and expression? As you identify the areas that you want to change, utilizing your value system, make sure your growth objectives resonate with your inner desires.

Sample Values Chart

Respect	Faith	Caring	Relationship	Health
Love	Forgiveness	Spirituality	Pleasure	Discover
Intensity	Adventure	Clarity	Balance	Joy
Learning	Fun	Gratitude	Wellness	Financial
Acceptance	Harmony	Fun	Service	Passion
Compassion	Beauty	Creativity	Learning	Self-Worth
Beauty	Order	Organization	Excited	Competent
Dependable	Respectful	Intelligent	Emotion	Responsible

5. **Develop a realistic plan of what it will take to accomplish these things.** Ask yourself, "What will it take for me to accomplish this task?" Many times we think that the task is bigger than it is. We need to break down any plan into bite-sized, easily accomplished pieces.

   Follow these steps to break down goals just as you would to prepare to do complex patient care. They are:
   1. Ask yourself, "What steps do I have to take to get the task accomplished?"
   2. Assign a time to complete each task. (i.e., January 30, 2010.)
   3. Consider what resources you might need to accomplish this task. Just like patient care, you need the proper tools to work with. (e.g., time, money, less time at work, a more stable schedule, etc.)
   4. Establish checkpoint goals along the way. What do you plan to have accomplished within 15 days, 30 days or 35 days of the actual goal.

6. **Choose two strategies to change at the same time.** Select two areas from your personal growth list to work on together. Many times we will attempt to achieve one area and leave the others because we are accomplishing something. It is imperative that you accomplish your goals in groups. When you create the space and time to complete your objectives, do all that you can in those moments.

7. **Get a buddy to run with.** If possible, hook up with a nurse friend who wants to achieve their own goals. Call one another weekly about your goals. Check in, weigh in and share what is working and what is not working. Share solutions.

8. **Get started!** Don't wait until Monday or until you get the right nursing shoes. You must act now. Things change so quickly in life that if you don't act today, you won't start. If you wait until tomorrow, you'll still be just as tired.

9. **Don't check results.** The point in this phase is to begin to identify some areas to improve the inner workings of your life. This does not mean that things are going to be perfect overnight. It does mean that you can immediately begin to move your life in ways that fulfill you instead of maintaining a life which is unfulfilling. If that means finding a job at a smaller hospital that affords you more time to enjoy your personal life, then so be it. You can still be a nurse and have a happy, fulfilling personal life in every facet.

The second stage of personal growth is MOTION

If you are in motion, you realize some of the areas of personal growth, but have not developed a consistent habit of achieving your goals. For example, you may play golf during the spring and summer but fail to add to the list during the winter and fall. The idea is that we understand that we want to continue the activities, events and energy that fuel us outside of work. As health care professionals, our work is demanding, and we need to release our tension with things which make us laugh, stimulate the mind and make us happy.

Understand there are eight areas of personal growth. When we are in motion we are usually accomplishing up to four areas of personal growth. Using the Wheel analogy, we are then able to move, but it is still a bumpy ride because there are other parts of ourselves we are not acknowledging.

It is my goal to see every person have the active ability to create a world that includes self-actualization. My friends have always been amazed by my ability to pursue my intellectual and spiritual growth whilst maintaining hobbies and special interests and pursuing good physical health. I am the perfect coach for you, because I know what it takes to make the time.

The strategies for Motion

1. **Date yourself in advance.** Plan a date in the future with yourself. Purchase tickets, make reservations or reserve the date with a friend to motivate yourself toward your goal. This might include going to the coffee shop to enjoy a warm drink, making a visit to the bookstore to read a magazine or enjoying a movie. Splurge and take in a concert. You decide: But decide you must.

2. **Put your self-commitments on a personal
   calendar.** When you make the commitment
   to yourself, make it official on your family's
   calendar as well as your personal calendar.
   Many times you can share your goals with other
   nurses and allied health professionals. Setting an
   example and providing motivation for others is a
   great way to force accountability.

3. **Get an accountability partner.** This could be
   a person with their own goals to accomplish,
   another nurse, or just a favorite friend who is
   pulling for you.

The last stage of personal growth is ACCELERATION

Acceleration permits nurses to soar. When we accelerate, we
are able to move forward with our dreams. Generally, we are
able to accelerate on that Wheel of Life as individuals. If you
are in a car with square wheels, how fast will you get to your
destination? Not very fast I should say. Well, the same is true
when we only cultivate two or four areas of our lives. At a
minimum, it is of great benefit to accomplish six to eight
areas of our lives. This allows us to have a smoother ride in
life. The reason is simple: Since we are connecting to and
acknowledging ourselves, we are able to move forward with
our dreams, plans and goals.

Simply by design we are under pressure from the time we pull
into the hospital parking lot until the time we lay our head on
the pillow at night at home. We often can't sleep because our
minds keep racing; our thoughts keep controlling our bodies.
This often leaves us with little time or energy for ourselves.

I have found if you want to ensure that you take care of your
interests each day, you have to place them at the top of the list.

This may sound selfish. However, I am not saying you should stop meeting the needs of your patients or the hospital. I am suggesting that if you don't put yourself first, then you will never accomplish anything for yourself. On the night before, plan the things you want to accomplish for yourself. Next, tell all necessary parties what you need from them. Don't be shy. Tell the nurse manager that you are unable to do a double shift on this day – and stick to it. Being clear about what you want to do will allow you to solicit the help of others.

Your goal is personal growth. Living a life void of growth is neither rich nor healthy. We want to be positive examples of success, and we can't be if we're living a life that does not reflect our hearts. A life that is rich with personal growth reflects the desires of our hearts.

The Strategies for Acceleration are:

1. **Continue to add to your list from the Nurture-Me Wheel. Be creative.**

2. **Ask yourself the following questions:** What are my personal visions, missions and passions? What are my goals?

3. **Create an affirmation or self talk statement that affirms you.** (i.e., I love how much energy I have when I exercise therefore, I will work-out three times a week)

The challenge for you is to take a good look at the life you have created and examine it thoroughly. Is this the life that you have planned, or is this the life that you have gotten by default? Making the decision to guide your life is the best way to ensure personal growth and success.

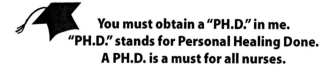

You must obtain a "PH.D." in me.
"PH.D." stands for Personal Healing Done.
A PH.D. is a must for all nurses.

The five top reasons to personally grow:

1. **You deserve it!** Take some time and write down why you deserve to be your best. What do you give your family and friends? What do you give to your patients?

2. **Others are watching your example of success!** Do they see a balance in your life?

3. **You want a better life!** Know that life is offering you more. You have gotten in the way of a life which you can enjoy. You want to be happy.

4. **Why not be happy!** Live a life that is satisfying.

5. **Personal growth will allow you to connect with yourself and figure out who you are!** Taking the time to get to know yourself will allow you to change the course of your life. I have clients who have accepted the demands of life believing that they are forever going to be unfulfilled, unexcited and unhappy. Why accept this as your reality when you can choose your life?

Earn a PH. D in Nurture-Me!

Chapter Objective:

• To identify specific areas for personal growth.

✎ Assignment 1:

Look at your life as it is and consider improving other areas on the Wheel of Life to enhance balance and wholeness.

1. Identify two areas in which you would like to personally grow:

2. What action can you take today to begin to realize growth in this area? (e.g., if the area is health: go to the gym or walk the perimeter of the lake for a minimum of 30 minutes three times a week...or schedule doctor visits with all physicians)

3. Over the next 30 days, what steps can you take to make your personal growth a priority?

4. What steps does your goal require to make it happen?

✎ Assignment 2:

Look at the Wheel of Life. Identify two areas that you would like to change *today.* Answer the following questions about those areas:

1. What do I want to accomplish in this area of my life?

2. What resources or requirements does this activity require to make it happen?

3. What are the possibilities once I make this change?

4. What are the benefits to me? My family? My friends?

Practices:

✓ Email your Nurture-Me Success Partner daily, weekly or bi-weekly depending on what you have decided. Let them know what action you have taken toward your goal.

✓ Take a minimum of 15 minutes each day to plan how you will accomplish your objective the next day.

Take a moment and let me know how you're doing! Go to www.findingdefinitions.com/caregivers.html!

_____

_____

_____

_____

_____

_____

_____

_____

_____

_____

_____

_____

_____

_____

_____

_____
_____
_____
_____
_____
_____
_____
_____
_____
_____
_____
_____
_____
_____
_____
_____
_____
_____
_____
_____
_____
_____
_____
_____
_____
_____
_____
_____

_____
_____
_____
_____
_____
_____
_____
_____
_____
_____
_____
_____
_____
_____
_____
_____
_____
_____
_____
_____
_____
_____
_____
_____
_____
_____
_____
_____

$\mathscr{F}$ Chapter 3
inding Time

Melissa works 60 hours a week. She wakes at 4 am and works until 7pm. She arrives for nurses' report at 6; 45 am at the hospital where she works. She is on her feet all day. She struggles with finding personal time to go to the gym, to run personal errands, and to pursue a personal passion. She has a nanny, but as usual, her work days are often occupied with meetings, physicians, unplanned interruptions and patient care. She longs for more flexibility.

Linda, is an ARNP who, works both day and night. She wakes up at 5:30 a.m. to prepare for the day. She works until 9:30pm every night Monday through Friday. She can't even go to the bathroom without being disturbed by one of the Medical Assistants asking her questions.

The purpose of this chapter is to help nurses find time for them-selves. As a busy person myself, I understand the specific strategies that nurses must employ to succeed. Unlike most time-management or organize-your-life self-help books, I will provide you with specific techniques created just for nurses.

As health care professionals, we have distinct challenges that consistently prevent us from finding personal time. Some of the challenges are self-inflicted, such as patient favoritism, fatigue, stress, and Super-Nurse mentalities, while others are external, such as unscheduled interruptions, changes in work schedules and therefore any personal schedule you may have designed. This chapter will shed some light on all of these challenges which are presented in the life of a nurse.

In previous chapters we have discussed your blueprint, the benefits of personal growth, how to assign your life meaning, and strategies on self-care solutions. Now that you are clear about your goals and have alleviated your distractions and eliminated self-defeating thoughts the next phase is finding time to self-accomplish.

Your day is hectic. No two days are exactly the same. Although we may have the same general events in our day, we are never quite sure what the day will hold. In the midst of a complex patient care project, you could get a call from the school nurse telling you to pick up your child from school. While attempting to read the chart of a very sick patient that was just admitted to your unit, you might get interrupted 10 times by the same belligerent physician who wants something NOW.

Symptoms of Imbalanced Life

Answer these questions honestly with the intention of getting some understanding about areas you want to change. Use your journal to detail your responses.

Nurture "Me" Assessment

Consider the following:
1. Are you overloaded at work? Do you juggle several important tasks at once completing a little of each?
2. Are you overcommitted after work? Are you signing up
for a host of activities because you feel obligated to do
these commitments?
3. Are you reactive? Are you always putting out the wildfires in

your personal life?

4. Do you feel there are never enough hours in a day?
5. Does your life lack planning?
6. Are your family activities driven by the words should and ought to?
7. Do you struggle with relaxation?
8. Do you feel you are the only person capable of doing a good job at _____?
9. Do you define yourself by doing for others?
10. Do you have trouble saying "No"?
11. Do you often find yourself doing things that you don't want to do?

If you have answered yes to four or fewer, then you are able to strike a balance in your life. If you have answered the affirmative to between five and eight, then you are in need of a balance makeover. If you marked over eight, then you are out of balance.

Steps To Creating More Balance

1. **Acknowledge that you are out of balance** (e.g., I am out of balance).

2. **Ask yourself the following, "What is making me feel out of balance?"** (e.g., I know that I am out of balance, because I work all the time and have very little time to enjoy life.)

3. **What does balance look like to you?** (e.g., Balance means that I can stop every day to simply enjoy a nice cup of tea)

4. **What resources do you have to help you manage balance in your life?** (e.g., friends,

other nurses who share common interests, a new acquaintance in the hospital cafeteria where you have your daily tea…)

5. **Which of these resources can you take ownership of today?** (e.g., I can make a commitment to do this at least once a day as soon as I get home from work)

6. **What is possible if you utilize this change?** (e.g., it's possible that I will feel more relaxed as I greet my family instead of being grumpy, snappy and irritated)

7. **Is this a change you would like to make?** Yes? Why?

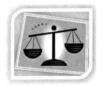 **It is unjust to not find time for yourself! You give to others, now start giving to you!**

A Nurse's Work Is Never Done

As nurses, we have a terrific opportunity to share in the joys, triumphs and wonders of our friends and patients. If you're like most nurses, you enjoy finding ways to become an active part of friendship and healing. Helping your patients get better both physically and mentally requires discipline, commitment, and love on your part.

As you meet the needs of your patients and responsibilities, you must find a way to meet your own needs as well. Have you ever considered doing something that meets your needs while you meet the needs of others? At this moment, I want you to dream about your ideal day on the unit. What would you be doing? Who would be there? How many patients would you have? How long would it last? Would it be exciting, or low-key? How would you make a difference in your life, as well as the lives of others?

What if I told you that you can create that dream life by making a few simple changes in your life? Would you believe me?

Too often as nurses we believe that our lives await us after we clock out and leave the hospital parking lot. What if I told you it is possible to enjoy your life today by simply making a few small steps?

Reflect on each of the following questions. Use your journal to answer.

Nurture "Me" Assessment

Consider the following:

1. What about my life makes me feel good?
2. How would patients and friends describe me?
3. What are my greatest accomplishments to date outside of the field of nursing?
4. How much of the day do I spend doing things to make myself happy?
5. What do I do for myself each day?
6. If I spent time doing only things that make me happy, what would I be doing?
7. If I only spent time with people who made me happy, who would that be?
8. How much fun do I want in my life?
9. What do I like to do to be happy?

Now that you have answered the questions above, you have an understanding of how out of balance you are and what your ideal life would look like. Now, look specifically at your actual days to create a plan to help you find time to do what you love.

Nurses: What are you doing all day besides giving of yourself to others?

Nurses have tons of activities that can go on the list of Contribution Activities. Contribution Activities are duties that have to be accomplished but don't necessarily leave a record of their successful completion. These are things you do not have to chart. These are the catch-all activities that go along with being a nurse, including:

Contribution Activities:

Responsibility	Tending to minor complaints	Reassuring families of patients
Being cordial	Staying calm in a crisis	Being cheerful no matter what
Listening	Fetching an extra cup of coffee for a patient	Checking safety
Organizing	Supervising Nurses Aides	Interacting with staff

🖉 Assignment 1:

Write down some of your most common Contribution Activities. They might include: reading a letter to a patient or wheeling someone down for a breath of fresh air. You name it. We all have them. Feel free to reference any of the activities above. Write them below or use your journal.

My Contributions:

1. _____

2. _____

3. _____

4. _____

5. _____

6. _____

You get the idea! Now, ask yourself what you can do for yourself while accomplishing these same contribution activities. This might mean that you will share your love of classical literature with a young patient who is scared, or that you will encourage a long-time elderly patient to walk with you so that you both can exercise. I call this blending.

What is blending?

Blending is when we combine personal objectives with nursing activity to self-accomplish. What I am suggesting is that we look for ways to blend ourselves into our lives.

Other examples include:

- While changing the dressing on a patient…talk about books you enjoy.

- While at work, consider creative ways to exercise alongside your patients. Consider helping

> another nurse catch up so they can leave on
> time, while you develop a friendship.

- For your lunch pack a brown bag - containing
  your favorite healthy snack, a new book,
  calendar or crossword puzzle.

- A patient is having a birthday, make a friend for
  you. It is possible to still make personal connections with others while you do your job.

- At home, assign a time for everyone to D.E.A.R.
  (Drop Everything And Read). This will give you
  some time to finish the book that you started at
  work.

The idea is to create opportunities to self-accomplish during
the activities that we naturally do as nurses and individuals.

As nurses, we have done the exact opposite. We don't seize
the opportunities to do anything for ourselves until the day
has officially ended. Many of us are still searching for that
extra time at the end of the day, week or years to do something for ourselves.

Taking this time to create a list of blending possibilities will
allow you to be playful and responsive to your own needs
while being of service to others. Bring yourself into the activities with your coworkers. With some of these activities, it's
tougher than others. But it is possible for all of these activities
to provide some level of support for ourselves as we continue
to support and nurture others.

How to Blend:

When blending, ask yourself the following questions:

1. What goal(s) would I like to accomplish? Do you have weight-loss goals, friendships to establish, hobbies, or a specific interests like hiking, golfing, cooking, etc?

2. Identify the amount of time and space necessary to achieve this objective. Does this goal have to be accomplished all at once, or is it possible to break it into bite-size portions?

3. Identify a place in your day where you can implement this objective. Is it possible to park a few blocks away from work and drop into that new shop you've wanted to check out when walking back to your car? Could you read a book during your lunch break? Can you share a good book with a coworker?

Examples of a Blended Life:

On the way home from work, instead of going straight home I go to my favorite neighborhood park where I can see the lake. I drive up close to the lake and I open my sunroof, play the soft music I love and read my favorite magazine or just watch the wildlife. For that hour I am transported, renewed and rested.

I work on a rehab unit and deal with patients who are in physical rehabilitation. I used to complain that I didn't have time to exercise like I wanted. A perfect opportunity presented itself when one of my patients had to go to dialysis three times a week. I wheel her down to the unit, and take the stairs back to the floor. Hiking up four flights of stairs three times a week has helped me meet that goal.

In the morning when I have my first cup of coffee as I get ready for work, I light a candle for me. I love the smell of aromatic candles. Now while I do something that I have to do in the morning to prepare for the day, I do something that transcends my environment.

Blending Opportunities

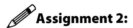 **Assignment 2:**

Write down what you can do for yourself for each of the activities that you identified from assignment 1. (Copy your contribution activities from assignment 1) Be creative. At first it might take you a minute because you never thought about doing any self-accomplishing task while fulfilling your responsibilities as a nurse. Be patient with yourself and give yourself time to Dream Big.

My Contributions	My Blending
1. _____	_____
2. _____	_____
3. _____	_____
4. _____	_____
5. _____	_____
6. _____	_____

Now commit to self-accomplishing! How many possibilities daily do you REALLY have in your busy schedule to include you?

Practices:

Take a snapshot of your typical day, and look for the possibilities to self-accomplish each day. Every day identify a minimum of one activity where you can possibly do something for both your patients and yourself at the same time.

Use the following chart to write down your daily schedule. Each week, update your schedule for the week to include any new activities. The purpose of this calendar activity is to make you aware of all you do. Don't be shy here. I want you to include everything you do to make your days happen. Too often we minimize the small activities such as making coffee, taking out the trash as you leave or stopping to pet the neighborhood mutt. This exercise will start by running the span of your week. Take some time and really think about how you spend your days. The purpose of the exercise is to help you see how you spend your days. Let's begin:

1. Under "Activity," indicate how you spend your time with coworkers and patients. Include any and all activities that you perform daily. Be sure and include the smallest, most minute things.

2. In addition, look at the time of day each of these activities is performed. Be specific.

3. Next, where are you performing these activities? In the patient rooms, at the nurses' station, or some other location?

4. Finally, list any possibility for you to do something for you with each activity.

Lorna Says: Do you see how blending can be accomplished such that one cohesive structure is made from two? Can you see how Mia and I have blended together to create a stronger support system for each other, and you?

Snapshot of your day

Monday

Activity	Time	Location	Blending Activity
i.e. Soccer Practice	*5:30–6:30pm*	*Soccer Field*	*Read a book in the car.*

Tuesday

Activity	Time	Location	Blending Activity

Wednesday

Activity	Time	Location	Blending Activity

Thursday

Activity	Time	Location	Blending Activity

Friday

Activity	Time	Location	Blending Activity

Saturday

Activity	Time	Location	Blending Activity

Sunday

Activity	Time	Location	Blending Activity

Promise yourself today you will incorporate "YOU" into your life.

Opportunities to incorporate ourselves into our lives are all around us. For nurses to self-accomplish, they need what is attempting to be created Taking this time to create different lists of blending possibilities will allow you to be "planful" and responsive to your needs as well as the needs of others.

Too often, I hear stories of nurses who go days, weeks, months or years putting themselves on hold. These people are looking for permission and the opportunity to enjoy their lives. Creating a list of possibilities for you makes it easier to find small ways to realize personal happiness every day.

The Benefits of Blending Your Life:

✓ Blending creates opportunities to enjoy your life daily.

✓ Blending is an efficient use of time.

✓ Blending gives nurses a new perspective when planning their day.

✓ Blending allows patients to see self-care in action.

✓ Blending helps health care workers find easy ways to incorporate themselves into their lives every day.

✓ Blending allows you to consciously acknowledge your needs and wants daily without putting yourself on hold.

✓ Blending gives nurses new options. It provides a new mindset for self-care.

Additional strategies on blending:

1. Make the things you enjoy easily accessible. Make your car your mobile university. Take your books on tape with you for your vehicle. Pack a book/magazine for just for you.

2. Joke with your coworkers. So often we tend to work and don't take the opportunity to have fun while we do it. Eat your lunch outside, read a book for you, or journal. As nurses, many times we keep every second of our day busy when we could look for opportunities to enjoy what is before us.

3. Make your home environment reflect the things that you love such as beautiful flowers, candles, or gardens.

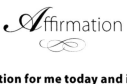

$\mathscr{A}$ffirmation

I took an action for me today and it felt great!

_____

(Your Signature)

_____
_____
_____
_____
_____
_____
_____
_____
_____
_____
_____
_____
_____
_____
_____
_____
_____
_____
_____
_____
_____
_____
_____
_____
_____
_____
_____
_____
_____
_____
_____

_____
_____
_____
_____
_____
_____
_____
_____
_____
_____
_____
_____
_____
_____
_____
_____
_____
_____
_____
_____
_____
_____
_____
_____
_____
_____
_____
_____
_____
_____

Chapter 4
Finding Meaning
Redefining and Creating Change in Your Life

Here are two examples of typical nurses:

Jane is a Registered Nurse who has realized a lot of professional success. She is known as a hard worker and is a top performer. She also has a family, consisting of her three children and her husband of seven years. She had a dream of becoming a caterer, a dream she felt was impossible. She felt that the demands of home and work would never allow her to do what she really wanted to do. Every year she talked about her love for catering with her family and friends. Everyone thought it was impossible because she worked 60+ hours a week on the unit at the hospital, Sso she decided to put her dreams on the shelf.

Paula has a work schedule better than most nurses. She works in a physician's office and is a very dedicated mom to her three children. She has managed to meet the needs of her children efficiently. She has enrolled her children in piano, tae kwon do, t-ball and gymnastics. As a wife she is equally committed. She manages to provide varied and balanced meals for her husband and children. She is considerate of her husband and makes sure that she and the children give her husband space and time to relax in the comfort of his home. She is always busy. She continues this way every day. One day seems to roll over into the next.

This is only half of the story…. what is missing?

What is missing from your life? What do you want for you? Do you still have dreams left to accomplish? What are they?

A Nurse's Work

Why is it that as nurses, we believe we have to sacrifice ourselves to be wonderful and effective contributors?

You've been on the plane before take off--the flight attendant instructs what to do in the event of an emergency. We are instructed to put on our air mask FIRST, before helping others. As nurses we should employ the basic self-life saving strategies of the airlines. The first thing a flight nurse is taught to do upon landing is assess the scene. Don't become part of the problem.

Let's talk about why this is important.

In order to truly help someone else you must begin by helping yourself. In order to truly be a wonderful contributor, you must help yourself FIRST.

Imagine that you are a cup which is always half-full or empty. Your cup is never full because you don't allow yourself the opportunity to replenish and renew. How can you then fill another cup?

When we give from a full cup we are kinder, nicer, more patient more creative and loving. Helping yourself first enables you to better help others.

Remember your Nurture-Me script? Well, your coworkers are watching your example of self-care and neglect. We would never tell our patients to self-sacrifice if we knew it would be to their detriment. Yet, we are teaching by example indirectly that we are not important.

Quite frankly, you deserve to do something for yourself because you give so much to the lives of everyone around you. As a personal coach, I encourage my clients to create a supportive network of friends and family, establish a work/life balance, and set personal boundaries.

Before I tell you how to "fill your cup," take a few moments to define your life in general. Find a quiet location, free of interruptions. Use your journal to detail your responses. It is important to be as open and honest with yourself while completing this exercise. Utilize these questions as a guide to get you to think about what your life means. There are no right or wrong answers; just insight into the areas that require more care.

Nurture "Me" Assessment

Consider the following:

1. What about my life make me feel good?
2. How would people describe me?
3. What are your greatest accomplishments to date?
4. How much time of the day do I spend doing things to make myself happy?
5. What do you do for yourself each day?
6. If you spent time doing only things that make you happy, what would you be doing?
7. If you only spent time with people that made you happy, who would that be?
8. How much fun do you want in your life?
9. What do you like to do to be happy?
10. Do you feel guilty when doing something for yourself? Yes   No   Why?
11. When did you last experience this guilty feeling? Describe the situation:
12. (Using the example from #11) What steps could you take to minimize your feelings of guilt?

Most nurses allow the emotions of guilt and shame to influence their life choices. We feel guilty about the things we have already accomplished but also for the things we have yet to accomplish. Have you ever made plans to go out with a friend as soon as your shift is over when, just before leaving, one of your favorite patients starts to decompensate? You immediately thought "Maybe I should not leave, because this person needs me." If you chose to leave anyway, I guarantee that you called the unit once or twice to make sure matters had not gotten worse, and you probably still felt guilty for leaving in the first place. Or, maybe whenever you think of doing something for yourself you simply feel selfish. Perhaps you are thinking that it is unfair for you to put any of your needs on someone else's agenda.

As health care professionals there are several things keeping us away from our dreams, plans and goals. Any time you want to make a change you must raise your standards.

In order to assign meaning and value to your life, you must:

✓ Define a clear vision for your life.

✓ Eliminate self-defeating habits that stop you in your tracks.

✓ Identify triggers that keep you from accomplishing your goals.

Defining a Clear Vision for Your Life

What do you want for you? Consider where you are right now and think about where you want to be. Maybe you want to pursue excellence in your physical health, or perhaps you want to be well traveled. Once you identify what you want, you can begin to make small changes or adjustments toward this vision.

What are your dreams? A dream is your personal ambition. The compositions of our dreams have many forms. The first are our mental images.

✎ Assignment 1:

Take a few moments to journal your responses. Read the following questions below. Close your eyes, and reflect before you respond.

1. What do you really want for your life?

2. What comes to your mind?

3. Are you envisioning peace and harmony, recreation, or that career you've always wanted?

4. What do you see for you?

5. How do these images make you feel? Relaxed, happy, anxious or excited?

This is a great exercise to start figuring out what you want for your life.

Perhaps you want to lose those extra pounds, or maybe you want to enroll in school for some graduate courses. Everything starts with a vision for your life. For example, once you decide that your personal health is a priority, you can then set the goal to lose 15 pounds. Next, you will take the necessary steps to achieve that objective by locating a local gym, by working out, or by identifying a person at work or in your community to walk or run with four times each week. It's that simple.

Ask yourself *how* you are going to accomplish your goal. The most important question to ask is *what* you plan to accomplish. Being clear on what to accomplish is the key to our success.

Changing our life takes commitment. It means that we have to overcome our fears, excuses, procrastination and our schedule to create the life we want. Many times we have to change the way we think and the way we behave to clear the way for the things we want.

Eliminating Self-Defeating Habits

Make a commitment with yourself that once you identify your vision for your life you will become partner with yourself in the process of change. We have to be our own instruments for change. We have to create the change we want by reinventing our behaviors. Bad habits keep us stuck in our old ways. We need to make different choices that aid our process to self accomplishment.

Reasons we stop what we start:

- We assume we already know the outcome of a new experience. Have you done this? You want to try something new and different but you presume to know what the new experience will bring.

- Labeling ourselves by saying things like "I'm not good at…"

- Over-generalizing any new experience to suggest that it is not good. For example, maybe you arranged a night out with some friends for the first time. Upon returning home you described the evening as a waste of time and said that the restaurant food lacked the quality of home.

- Blaming others for what we have not done for ourselves.

- Comparing ourselves to others. When we do this we always compare our weaknesses to the strengths of others.

The idea here is to begin to make conscious choices. Think about what you want to accomplish, and choose to honor your desires with an action every day. Identify and remove thoughts from your mind which are defeatist. If we want to change our lives, we must change our old self-defeating patterns. We must begin by believing we deserve that which we the desire. Many times we don't believe we deserve every thing we are trying to accomplish.

Align yourself with the possibility of success!

Identifying the triggers that keep you from accomplishing your goals

A series of events could change at any moment when we try to self-accomplish. In an instant, policies at the hospital could change to patient focus and the workload could seem impossible. To self-accomplish, you need to be proactive. Account for these looming unscheduled interruptions. For example, have you ever attempted to read a book and yet never managed to read even one page? What happened? Asking yourself this important question can help you anticipate what your most common distractions are so that you can plan for them.

Triggers are simply distractions. You may find that you are at home loading the dishwasher after dinner and attempting to listen to an audio presentation that is needed for your CEU's, your children begin to disagree and argue, distracting you from listening to the presentation.

Recognizing all common distractions whether at work or at home is important, because it clarifies what you need to change in your day to self-accomplish. Ask yourself: "How can I overcome this obstacle, situation or distraction?" If the children fight when you unload the dishwasher, why not propose a time to Drop Everything And Read – DEAR - for the children after dinner? This will allow you to complete part of your audio presentation and give the children a task to accomplish.

Kelly's daughter, Stacy, always wanted her mom whenever Kelly attempted to read a book. I taught Kelly this simple technique called mirroring with her 18 month old. Instead of sneaking away to read, Kelly made reading a two-person activity, one she explained to Stacy. "We're going to read for 15 minutes. This is my book. Go get your Elmo book so you can read, too."

Stacy got her Elmo book and sat down next to Kelly. After a few minutes, Stacy put her book down and climbed into her mother's lap.

"No, not yet," Kelly said. "Reading time isn't over. You can get another book if you like, but we're going to read some more."

Stacy got another book. The first time Kelly tried the technique, she had to keep sending Stacy back for books; but, after a while, Stacy caught on.

Ted works 7am-7pm at St. Christopher's Regional Medical Center in Minnesota. He pushes himself from the time he arrives until the time he leaves. His only time to relax is during his short lunch break. After the arrival of a new nurse on the floor, Ted found that he was unofficially charged with her orientation to the floor. His phone would ring with questions ranging from the location of supplies to new floor admissions. Finally, Ted explained to the new nurse that he was on his break, and for her to ask someone presently on the floor. Although the new nurse seemed put off a bit at first, she got the idea and Ted's break time continued peacefully.

✎ Assignment 2: Complete the distraction log.

When do I most often have distractions? What am I doing? How long do they last?

Right now, I want you to write down 10 ways that you become distracted at home. Consider different times of the days and during different kinds of activities.

Activity (What are you doing?)	Distraction (What is the distraction?)	Time of the Day (Breakfast, Dinner, cleaning, etc.)
1.		
2.		
3.		
4.		
5.		
6.		
7.		
8.		
9.		
10.		

Mirroring Steps

- Talk with others and tell them the activity that you plan to accomplish and the amount of time it will take.
  - Stan is going to spend the next thirty minutes charting.

- At home, have your children mirror your activity. Teach your young children initially in one-, three- and five-minute intervals until they understand this activity.
  - Stacy is going to write on her pad for 15 minutes.

- Remember to be patient and kind but consistent while reinforcing your responsibilities.
  - I am still charting, but I will be happy to help you when I'm finished.

- Reward others when you are finished. Go help your coworker just like you promised, and ask if there is anything else you can assist with before you get busy again.

As nurses, we have to be proactive to include ourselves into our days. Taking the time to list your most common distractions will assist you in finding reasonable ways to self-accomplish in the company of your children.

Now you understand what you need to do to create the mindset for change in your life. Change requires us to redefine our priorities.

Do you recall the nurses that were mentioned previously? Well, Jane, the R.N., learned that if she wanted to have a catering business she could. She began to schedule herself into her life a few hours a week. She accomplished something for her business every week. She went from believing that she had no time to plan events, to planning three events. The largest event was a wedding with more than 200 guests.

Paula learned to set-some personal boundaries with her children. She put her children to bed at 8:00 pm, so she had some down time after a day of giving. In addition, she asked her husband if he would support her taking some time to take piano lessons. She can now read music and play the piano.

Both of these nurses used the techniques taught in this book to accomplish their once impossible goals. It's all about your clarifying the changes you want in your life. It is possible, and your friends and family love you and will accommodate your wishes. Just ask!

Strategies for developing a clear vision for your life and redefining your dream

1. Develop a clear vision for your life and redefine your dream.

2. Look at where you are and where you want to go next. Then begin to make small adjustments to propel you toward your goal. Stay committed to what you want by applying this book's lessons and by reviewing your journal.

3. Remember to eliminate self-defeating habits. If you want a different outcome, then do something different. Don't expect to achieve a different result if you continue to do the same things.

4. Identify the triggers preventing you from achieving your objectives. Become the expert of

your life. Figure out what are your reoccurring interruptions that get you off track. Be proactive and solution-oriented.

5. The goal is to create a life you love.

6. Increase your standards for living.

7. Dream big for your life. You deserve it. Create a life that is rich with personal fulfillment and self-connection.

8. Change unhelpful belief patterns. Get rid of thoughts that say you cannot take care of yourself and still be a good mother. These are untrue. Instead, look for ways to:
   ✓ Develop new strategies for change.
   ✓ Create a new way to live that reflects your values.
   ✓ Create your dreams, plans and goals by applying my strategies to make the changes that will help redefine your life.

You can have the life you want. Remember that self care is not negotiable, but necessary to be the best person possible. Yes, you can!

Nurses are always hungry and love to eat! Consequently, they are always looking for great recipes to make the perfect meal. Here is the recipe for enhancing your life esteem or assigning your life meaning.

Ingredients:
 courage   commitment
 big dreams   solutions
 goals

Preparation:

1. Set your temperature to the highest setting. In other words, have an open mind and heart.

2. Look at where you are and where you want to go next. Then, begin to make small adjustments to propel you toward your purpose.

3. Stay committed. To avoid losing focus, state your goals every day. Journaling your feelings and progress always helps.

4. Watch out for self defeating habits. If you want a different outcome, then do something differently.

5. Be aware of the triggers that keep you from achieving your objectives. Be proactive about finding solutions to the distractions that get you off track.

Yield:
 A healthy serving
 of a life you love!

Practices:

Identify your goals. Expand your list of goals from your exercises in the personal growth chapter. Look at more areas of your life that you want to change, (e.g., physical, social, intellectual, financial, spiritual). Identify two or three goals for each of these areas. Make your goals Believable, Achievable and Time Measurable. Goals should be clearly and simply stated. For example, I will eat healthy food at each meal of the day. When establishing goals, be specific and assign a time that identifies when you achieve this goal. Most importantly, commit to your goals. Mark your calendar every day you have worked toward your goal.

Please let me know how you are progressing by going to www.findingdefinitions.com/caregivers.html!

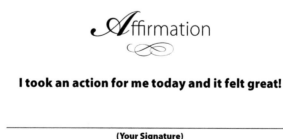

*A*ffirmation

I took an action for me today and it felt great!

_____
(Your Signature)

_____
_____
_____
_____
_____
_____
_____
_____
_____
_____
_____
_____
_____
_____
_____
_____
_____
_____
_____
_____
_____
_____
_____
_____
_____
_____

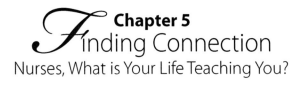

Chapter 5

Finding Connection
Nurses, What is Your Life Teaching You?

Pretend your life is a mirror. Your life is a mirror of your emotional and social health, your physical strength or weakness, your interests and favorite pastimes. What does your personal mirror reflect? Answer the following questions to help you see your reflection. Use your journal to detail your responses:

Nurture "Me" Assessment

Consider the following:

1. Who are your closest friends? When did you last spend three hours or more with these friends?
2. What are your hobbies? How much time have you spent doing these?
3. When was the last time you saw a play or concert for you?
4. Do you like your wardrobe? What looks good on you?
5. How do you relax? What do you enjoy doing at home?
6. Do you like your body? What is your favorite physical trait? Which traits would you like to change?
7. Are you happy? What is the evidence of your happiness?
8. What do you like about yourself? What makes you special?
9. Name one item in your home that is just for you. How often do you get to enjoy this item?
10. What do you love about your life? When do you experience this?
11. What must you change about your life?

12. Are you getting enough rest? What time do you go to bed? What time do you wake each day?
13. How is your diet?
14. What other questions do you need to ask yourself?

When you see yourself in your life mirror, do you see the life you envisioned? As nurses, we forget to think about our lives while we tend to the lives of others. Remember, although it is a wonderful experience to make a difference in the lives of others, it is your life too.

Nursing is a process of giving, loving and celebrating. It can also be heartbreaking and full of disappointments as well. Choosing to be health care professionals who celebrate the roles and responsibilities involved, we must, at the same time, realize that this is not enough to complete us.

Being a nurse does not completely define us, but enhances what already is. For example, if you are healthy, then you have the opportunity to share that piece of you with your patients. If you have a supportive network of friends and family, then you are able to teach others the benefits of being loved by a world that is bigger than you. This shows you recognize the benefits of trusting and sharing with others.

Dan, a nurse and single father of two children between the ages of three and eight, was too tired to encourage his children to go to after school activities. He vowed to get more energy. He made the decision to connect through exercise each morning before work. He walked at 5:00am with one other neighbor. After two months, he formed a neighborhood walking club. Today, Dan is 20lbs lighter and has consistent opportunities to share with friends and exercise.

Now, Dan encourages his children to participate in soccer and basketball activities to promote their own physical fitness.

Whatever your reflection, you will share that with your patients, coworkers, and children. If your reflection is one of frustration, disappointment and regret, guess what? You will share those also. So now is your opportunity to learn to appreciate your reflection of love, respect, admiration, acceptance and nurturing. A reflection is powerful because it shows us who we really are. Who are you really? What defines you?

The reflection questions are provided to help you connect with yourself. Many nurses have not taken the time to ask themselves important and relevant questions about how they connect to the essentials of living. Often I speak with health care professionals who have no sense of connection to themselves. They want to know which questions to ask themselves. Using these powerful and necessary questions will guide you towards self-connection.

The Results of the Lack of Connection:

Inability to feel
Unable to identify preferences
Confusion about personal choices
Feeling overwhelmed about making decisions
Afraid of failure or the unknown
Overly analytical about choices
Clueless
Insecure

Let's start changing those feelings.

🖋 Assignment 1: Reflections.

Write in the space below, or use your journal.

First ask yourself, "What do I like about myself?" Write down what you like about the following:

Physical features (Lorna Says: Blank spaces are not allowed.) Consider your favorite physical attributes.

List your physical favorites from you best traits to your least favorite.

1. _____

2. _____

3. _____

4. _____

5. _____

Relationships

What type of friend are you? To answer this question look at your closest friendships. How would you describe your closest friendships? How would your friends describe you as a friend?

List your friendship attributes from your best traits to your least favorite.

1. _____

2. _____

3. _____

4. _____

5. _____

Hobbies

What activities do you enjoy? When answering this question, consider the activities that you currently enjoy. If you are struggling here, then consider the activities that you enjoyed in your past.

List your activities from your favorite to the least favorite.

1. _____

2. _____

3. _____

4. _____

5. _____

Finding Time

When was the last time you did something for yourself?

When answering this question, think about how you feel when doing something for yourself. Do you feel guilty, selfish or frivolous when you take time for you?

List the activities that you do for yourself from your favorite to the least favorite.

1. _____

2. _____

3. _____

4. _____

5. _____

Physical appearance:

List the last time that you bought new clothes Do you know what looks great on you? Sometimes as nurses we say that we are going to wait until we shed unwanted pounds, or start working out before we invest in an outfit that makes us look great. Many times we struggle with the practicality of splurging for ourselves. Is this you?

When was the last time you purchased new clothes? What were they? Where did you get them? When did you wear them last?

1. _____

2. _____

3. _____

4. _____

5. _____

Now that you have completed this exercise, you have an idea of what your life is reflecting to you. Your life may be reflecting a greater need for personal space or quiet time. Perhaps your life is reflecting a desire to connect socially with friends or establish meaningful hobbies. The goal of any reflection is to learn to love and appreciate what you see. Do you like what you see?

As your coach, I want to help you enhance your view of you. When you look at yourself I want you to love what you see, respect your limits and appreciate your gifts.

Here are five steps to consider when looking at your reflection:

Visualize your best self when looking at your reflection. Visualize yourself as productive, loving and caring. Remove the limiting self-defeating obstacles that keep us stuck and encumbered.

Initiate the change you want. Begin with action! Start today to implement some of your favorites from your reflection list. Use this list over and over to give you a guide of the new things that you want to enhance your life today.

Encourage yourself with words of acceptance and affirmation Use words that make you feel victorious instead of language that leaves you feeling hopeless. Write down positive affirmations about your reflection and post them on a 3 X5 note cards.

Work the plan. Create a plan of action to enhance your view of you.

Self Connection

When you take the time to self-connect, you create a space in your life to hear from your inner desires. What are the desires of your heart? What do you really want?

When you spend your days fielding the requests of those who direct your days, how do you self-connect?

You must employ the following strategies to self-connect as a nurse and individual. They are:

1. Assign a space in your home as a **Connection Place.** A connection place is a place where you can go uninterrupted every day. This could be your favorite sofa by the window in your living room or it could be a vanity that reflects your beauty. A connection place creates a place in your home that fuels you and fills you. This is your home get-away. Most importantly, it is your physical symbol/representation of peace at home.

2. Meet in that connection space a minimum of 15 minutes each day. I believe every person deserves peace in their life daily. At a minimum, 15 minutes.

3. Equip your space with your tools. Your tools are the following: *Finding Time to Care for Me: The Nurse's Guide to Self-Care* journal, special music, visual pictures that motivate you toward your goal. Your tools will prove an invaluable resource because by creating these 15 minutes to connect with yourself daily you will discover who you are. This book will be your best friend as you do the work necessary to redefine who you are.

During the time that you spend in your connection place, you will slowly discover who you are. You will better hear your voice, and you will plan time for yourself into each day. My goal for you is for you to be present in your life every day. You will no longer be in a quandary on how to include yourself in every area of your day.

You will become a nicer person to those who care about you. You will become better able to love because you love yourself. You will become a better nurturer and nurse because you will truly have nurtured yourself. Essentially, I am saying that learning who you are will enable you to present your best self to anyone you come in contact with.

We have had it all mixed up. We have expected nurses to balance the impossible with a smile. The reason I excel is because I excel as a person. When I am in the company of others, I am whole; not scattered, fragmented or broken. What about you? What if it were possible to enjoy your life consistently? What if you did not have to have bad days - or days when the chaos of work made you crazy- because you had a handle on you?

I have always consistently found ways to pursue my happiness every day no matter the company I share. This process taught me how to be peaceful, loving, respectful, whole, funny, and spontaneous.

It's All About Self-Connection

When we create a space in our lives to hear from our inner desires, we set the framework for something great. Taking a moment to get quiet every day or every evening will provide us with the time to think about and consider new possibilities and opportunities.

What is your something great? What types of connections do you want to see at work in your life?

Defining your life is a commitment that takes courage and clarity. I am glad you have decided to find your personal definitions. As you embark on this journey of self-care, self-fulfillment and self-connection, you will find personal definition. Too often, as health care professionals, we become so involved with the cares, concerns and demands of others that we forget what we want. This program was created to aid you in staying connected through your professional and individual experiences and reconnect if you have lost sight of you.

Practices:

Track your self-connection. Ask yourself the following questions daily, weekly and monthly to see if you are on track. There is no right or wrong choice. You know what you want to create from the assessment. Do your answers line up? If not, you have some work to do. If so, then good for you! You are taking the time to get to know you again and maintaining that connection.

1. Self-connection is _____ .

2. I self-connect (once- twice- three) times a week.

3. I go to the _____ in my home, office or _____ to self-connect.

4. I self-connect_____ minutes for the day. My goal is _____ minutes per day.

5. My idea of connecting with myself involves ___ _____ .

6. I feel _____ when I
   take the time to connect with myself.

7. Self-connecting daily has helped me _____
   _____ .

8. I spend _____ amount of time with myself
   each week.

$\mathcal{A}$ffirmation

I took an action for me today and it felt great!

_____

(Your Signature)

_____

_____

_____

_____

_____

_____

_____

_____

_____

_____

_____

_____

_____

_____

_____

_____

_____

_____

_____

_____

_____

_____

_____

_____

_____

_____

_____

_____

_____

_____

_____

_____

_____

_____

_____

_____

_____

_____

_____

_____

_____

Chapter 6
Finding Solutions

Nurses are always looking for the best solutions to solve life's problems. As it relates to self-care, the greatest challenge is our own defunct ideology that says it's impossible to be a great caregiver yet personally grow.

Recently, at a workshop I conducted in Atlanta, participants spoke honestly about their challenges in finding time, growing personally, finding connection, and sharing their "Me" blueprint for self-accomplishing.

Many health care professionals admit they place their own unrealistic standards of perfection on their spouses, child-care providers and other support-givers. Do you share these tendencies? What unrealistic standards have you set which limit the amount of support you can receive?

Many health care professionals have asked if there is one simple way of attaining self actualization. Many health care professionals have been running on auto-pilot for so long, they don't know how to get out of the vehicle. They have a difficult time seeing what the other possibilities might be for their lives. Is this you?

As I listened to these health care professionals, I immediately thought what nurses want are solutions to this very deeply emotional challenge of letting go in order to experience a new life. This chapter was created to give you some simple strategies to begin to create a new mindset.

To embrace a new perspective:
1. Raise your standards
2. Change your belief system
3. Change your strategy

Raise Your Standards

Anytime you want to make a change in your life you must first raise your standards.

Write down a list of the things that you are merely tolerating. Tolerations are things that we may or may not choose to change, but it is important to articulate what these things might be.

Some examples of things you might be tolerating as a nurse are:
- Degrading treatment from physicians
- Psychological abuse from patients
- No help from family to run the household

Lorna Says: Carry a small writing pad with you at all times, and jot down examples of things you tolerate so they are fresh. Use your journal to detail your responses.

Nurture "Me" Assessment

Consider the following:

1. What are you tolerating?
2. How might you modify these tolerations?
3. What are the benefits of making this change?

Changing What You Believe Is Possible

As nurses, we tend to believe that we cannot take care of ourselves and still take care of those in our charge. That simply is not true. We tend to believe that self-care means that we are selfish and somehow neglectful towards our responsibilities—another untruth. If you want to change your life, you have to be open to change. Many times, nurses will experience the symptoms that can hinder—or trigger—change in our lives, such as:

- Feeling run down
- Depressed
- Sadness
- Sickness
- Aches and pains

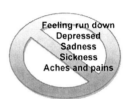

Making the decision to change will bring greater physical and emotional health.

Change Your Strategies

If we want to change our lives, we must change our old self-defeating patterns. We must begin by believing we deserve that which we desire. Many times we don't believe we deserve the very thing we are trying to achieve. We also have to stop tolerating the things that keep us from what we want. Some of the things we are wrong to tolerate are: lack of respect and appreciation, lack of personal time, lack of boundaries, financial constraints and an unfair household division of labor.

Communicate deliberately. Learn to say no – decisively. If you can't do it, just say you can't do it, and leave no room for negotiating. All too often we say, *"I might, well, possibly, um, we'll see. I'll call you tomorrow."* This allows the discussion to remain unresolved and open-ended.

Instead, practice delivering closing statements while looking in the mirror.

"No, I'm not going to be able to do that. Sorry."
"No, I'm not sure when I can."
"I'm sorry, but you can't bring her over today. It's not a good time."
"I'm sorry, I can't work overtime tonight: I have plans."
"You know, I'd love to help you, but that's not going to work."

Now you understand what you need to do to create the mindset for change in your life. Changing requires us to redefine our priorities.

The goal is to establish a personal vision and goals to complement that vision. Ask yourself what this objective requires of me, in order to accomplish it daily, weekly or monthly.

A terrific strategy to help nurses create solutions in their lives and make room for accomplishing goals is to employ what I call DIPP.

DIPP Stands For:
Delegate, Incorporate others, Plan, and Purge

Delegate some of your responsibilities at work to a Nurse's Assistant or GN when you can. I have found when we teach by delegation, they are willing participants. This applies at home as well; spouses are also more willing to help when they know what is expected of them.

1. What are some activities / responsibilities that you can delegate?
2. To whom can you delegate in your family?
3. What are some good reasons to delegate?

4. What are the benefits of delegating work responsibilities?
5. What new possibilities will you have when you delegate a task?
6. How does your environment benefit?

Incorporate others in your space. Create a support network for yourself. This network can include friends, family, coworkers, and others. Many times I have exchanged services with a friend. My friend and I switch watching each other's children five hours each week. She watches my son for two and half hours on Tuesdays and Thursdays, and I watched her child on Fridays so that she and her husband can spend time together. You can do this too. The idea is that no matter how hectic your schedule, you can always find time to Nurture-Me.

What creative ways can you incorporate others into your space?

List the names of either people or services that you can add to your space. Some examples might include: Friends, Relatives, and coworkers. (An 11, 12 or 13-year-old Mother's Helper could come over and watch your children to give you some time on the treadmill on your day off. They would have fun doing it, and that very small task would give you a half hour or 45 minutes extra time for yourself!)

1. What type of support do you need?
2. Which of these resources of support are available to you right now?
3. What are the possibilities for you when using this support?
4. What are the benefits to your family?
5. What does your ideal support system look like?

Plan

Plan your days in advance. Look for ways to incorporate your pleasures into what you will be doing. Pack a bag ahead of time for you – with your favorite snacks and something to do on your break. Take some of your favorite treats into work and when one of the Nurse's Assistants does a good job, reward them with a smile and a treat!

Plan each day at a minimum the night before. Consider the following:

1. What does your ideal day look like?
2. What resources are necessary for you to plan effectively?
3. What is possible for you when you plan?
4. What is the benefit to your family when you plan?

Purge

This is my favorite step. Purging is getting rid of the unnecessary. I used to drive my children all over to baseball and soccer practices and gymnastics, until I noticed they didn't really *like* baseball, soccer and gymnastics. I realized when the sign-up sheet came home from school, I asked them, "You want to take soccer, don't you?" And they'd grunt "Yeah. Okay." So we developed a new rule: If you want to do something, express yourself. Just tell Mom and Dad, and you can do those things, but if you don't bring it up, I'm not going to bring it up either. And it's not because I want to deny my children any kind of activity. It's because I have come to the realization that not everything is necessary.

No one benefits from purging more so than do nurses, as it helps free up precious time and energy which are such scarce commodities.

What can you get rid of in your schedule? What can you move to next week? Are there items on your list of things to do that could be eliminated? *(If it is not something that I need to do in the next 24 hours, then maybe it can be eliminated.)*

1. What can you eliminate from your day?
2. What are the personal benefits of purging this activity?
3. What are the benefits to your family?
4. What do your need to do to rid yourself of this life item? Make a call or say no working massive amounts of overtime.

When we DIPP we add more time and opportunity to achieve our goals.

Finally, here are some simple strategies that can help us find time for ourselves every day.

1. **Renew your mind.** Take some time every day to focus on something that makes you feel good. Eliminate things, events and people that drain your mental energy.

2. **Journal your feelings.** This is a wonderful way to keep a written record of your life. When I journal, I am often surprised by how much I am a creature of habit.

3. **Create a book or bulletin board with pictures of your dreams, plans and goals.** The goal is to give yourself visual reminders of the things you would like to accomplish. Some examples might be tickets to a favorite concert or lecture or a picture of a book you would like to finish reading. Place your book or board in your

connection place, the place that you go every day to be with you. Make it convenient.

4. **Give yourself a break every day.** Take a minimum of 15 minutes for yourself every day. This might require your getting up early or staying up later. It's worth it! You're worth it! Use this time to unwind and be empty. Try not to think about anything specific.

5. **Self-Accomplish in mouse bites.** Whatever you are trying to accomplish, remember that inch by inch it's a cinch; but, yard by yard it's hard. Take small steps toward your goals. The most important objective is to take small pieces *consistently.*

Some of you are saying it has been so long since I have thought about what I want. What would give you a great quality of life? Start by asking yourself, what do I value? I value quiet and reflection. As you clarify what you value, you will slowly be able to discover how to create peace within.

Maintenance

The objective of this book is to put you on a path to self-definition as an individual. Just like establishing any routine, it is equally important to identify a maintenance routine to self accomplish. I recommend the following:

1. Define a daily routine.
    - Visit your connection place daily.
    - Establish consistent times to plan daily.
    - View your daily calendar at a glance.
    - Keep a journal of progress.

2. Establish Nurture-Me Success Partners
   - Identify five accountability partners. They can be friends or other nurses you have met at work or your personal coach. Visit www.findingdefinitions.com/caregivers.html for these resources.
   - Establish consistent meeting times to consult with your partner or start Nurture-Me Club. Go to www.findingdefinitions.com/caregivers.html for details.

When you do these things you will become stronger than ever by not neglecting yourself.

Practices:

✓ **Observe your Physical Appearance.**
   Evaluating Physical Appearance
   1. Create a realistic wish list for change.
   2. Record the things that you love about yourself.

✓ **Date Yourself**
   1. Write down five things you want to do alone.
   2. Assign a date to accomplish these goals.
   3. Journal your successes and obstacles.

✓ **Dressing for success**
   1. Lose the hippie jeans. Stop wearing scrubs on your days off.
   2. Evaluate your wardrobe. Ask a fashionable friend for help
   3. Purge anything you haven't worn in a while or is ill-fitting.
   4. Plan your look.

✓ **What is under your skin?**
  1. Schedule a complete physical yearly.
  2. Visit the dentist yearly.
  4. Follow-up with specialist if you have any problems.

When you complete these actions you will be ready to love yourself again. These are simple solutions that will help you find personal definition.

Lorna Says: Understanding that self-love is the key to being able to live a full and happy life is paramount. If you care about yourself first, you are then able to care for others in a more honest, open fashion.

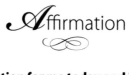

$\mathscr{A}$ffirmation

I took an action for me today and it felt great!

_____
(Your Signature)

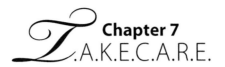

Chapter 7
T.A.K.E.C.A.R.E.

Now that you have experienced my program for creating a meaningful and fulfilling life, I want you to TAKECARE using my easy strategies for always considering your own needs.

Here are some reasons you need to T.A.K.E. C.A.R.E. of you:

1. Your life matters. You don't have to wait until the children graduate from high school or start nursery school to do something for yourself. Start today. Take small steps. Ask yourself: *What do I want? What do I like?*

   There is a saying, *"Never put off until tomorrow what you can do today."* If you enjoy it today, you can do it again, tomorrow.

   That's exactly my point. Begin to enjoy your life today.

2. It is possible to self-accomplish and be a great nurse and individual. Dispel the rumors that nurses can't find greatness for themselves and still take care of other demands in life. It is simply not true. You can carve out a slice of your life and do something consistently for you each week. Schedule a massage, a lunch with

coworkers at the hospital, or planting flowers in your yard. When we do something for ourselves consistently, we are renewed and rejuvenated.

3. Are you seeking a balanced life? Think about what it takes to balance on a balancing beam. First, you have to step onto the beam. Second, you must see where you want to go. Next, you will probably extend your arms to help you stay steady. Finally, you begin by taking small steps until you arrive at the end of the beam. Balancing any aspect of our lives requires focus, consistency, a total commitment and perseverance. If you want a life which includes your family, spirituality, financial goals and personal passion, then creating balance is your only option. When attempting to create balance in your life, you have to get started and consider what you want to accomplish. Scrutinize all areas in your day and take small steps until you get there.

4. Are you running on empty? Do you have more things to do than energy left to pull them off? Stop the roller coaster and understand that Super-Nurse is not real.

5. Enhance your standards and expectations. Elevate the way you live. Decide today you deserve the best.

6. Reduce your stress by learning to say *"No"*.

7. Establish boundaries and work to enforce them.

T.A.K.E.C.A.R.E.

Time. Make time for yourself in your life. What are your dreams, plans and goals? What do you still want to accomplish? As health care professionals, it is expected that we make time for work and family activities; yet, we forget to make time for ourselves. When was the last time you did something for you? How are you enriching your life? Are you fulfilled? When was the last time you planned a brown bag picnic for your lunch break at work with other nurses?

Arrange your days. As nurses, we can include ourselves into our days by planning the night before. When was the last time you completed reading a book? Make the things you enjoy easy to access. Make your car your mobile university. Take books on tape with you in your vehicle and catch up on your CEU's while stuck in traffic.

Keep your life simple. Are you overscheduled? Do you find you are running – everywhere and not able to enjoy the view? Why not? What is the race? Ask yourself, *"What activities can I eliminate from my life?"*

Evaluate your health. When was the last time you went to the doctor? When did you last go to your primary care physician or the dentist? I had a client – a well-educated person – who was shocked, upon visiting the dentist, to find that she had a broken tooth. She had never even noticed that her tooth was broken. What about you? What do you need to learn about your body? How is your emotional health?

Create a supportive network. Establish relationships with friends, family, coworkers, and friends of coworkers. Outsource your laundry and housecleaning, if possible. Create opportunities to ease your workload to reduce personal stress and anxiety during the workday. Ask others to help you. Solicit the help of family members, friends and neighbors.

Arrange a date with you. Yes, with you. Get to know yourself again. What are your hobbies and interests? What do you enjoy doing? Tell a story.

Relax every day. Give yourself a break every day. Stop the rollercoaster of life, and be still to hear your inner voice. Allot time in your days to relax at home. I suggest you create a quiet space in your home for relaxation and renewal.

Erase your need for perfection. You don't have to be perfect to have an enjoyable life. The house, the yard, the flowers, you – none of that has to be just perfect. Give your life the needed flexibility.

Being a nurse is signing up for a life of service, but not as a servant.

At home, are all of your family members helping with the housework? Arrange a meeting and coordinate the chores. Children under 10 should be provided a list for checking off their to-dos. Many times a nurse's feelings of being overwhelmed and under-appreciated are a toxic combination which will make you feel resentful over time. Stop and think: If everyone on the nursing unit worked completely independently outside of a cohesive goal, there would be chaos, wouldn't there. Teach your children to contribute to the family unit.

Remember you do matter and that your self-care is not negotiable, but necessary to be the best person possible.

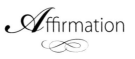

I took an action for me today and it felt great!

_____

(Your Signature)

_____

_____

_____

_____

_____

_____

_____

_____

_____

_____

_____

_____

_____

_____

_____

_____

_____

_____

_____

_____

_____

_____

_____

_____

_____
_____
_____
_____
_____
_____
_____
_____
_____
_____
_____
_____
_____
_____
_____
_____
_____
_____
_____
_____
_____
_____
_____
_____
_____
_____
_____
_____
_____
_____

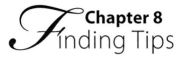

Chapter 8
Finding Tips

This bonus section was created as my gift to you. This is an assortment of newsletter articles I have written that will inspire you to change, using my simple strategies. Read and savor them. You will begin to see the key to rediscovering yourself is taking small steps. Be sure to become part of my mailing list. Sign up at.www.findingdefinitions.com/caregivers.html.

Nurse, do you know you?

Remember the song from the movie *Mahogany?* The song went, "Do you know where you're going to? Do you like the things that life is showing you? Do you get what you're hoping for? When you look behind you, are there no open doors. Do you know?"

This month, let's discuss your plans for your life. What are they? I bet if I asked you to tell me your family's plans for the month, you could come up with a host of activities. In addition, you probably know the list of to-do's that each person needs to accomplish as well. What about you? What are your plans? What are you going to do when you grow up and become a nurse?

Now is the time for you to answer these questions. As nurses, we often forget to dream for ourselves. Many times we ride on the dreams of our patients and workmates and forget that we can dream a real dream for us. When we work toward a goal, it fuels and fills us. It gives us a new sense of purpose.

Also, it sets an example for anyone who cares to watch – demonstrating we can self-accomplish and be still nurturing and loving.

Have you ever said to yourself that you were going to go back to school or pursue a new interest when you get the time? When that time arrives, you find that you have forgotten what it was that was once important to you. This is why as a health care provider you must not delay, but must decide what you want to do with-in your life now. Here are five steps to help you act today:

1. Write down five things that you want to do with-in your life. Remove all self-imposed imitations, and dream BIG!

2. What does each of these goals require? (For example, to earn your BSN, or attend graduate school, you might need to take evening or weekend courses.)

3. List five reasons that you think this idea won't work. Answer the following questions for each obstacle:
   • How can this opportunity work?
   • What do you have to overcome to accomplish this? (Do you need a more flexible schedule, financing, or is it purely motivation?)

4. What are the benefits? What will you gain by venturing into this new experience? Will you make new friends, learn something new, or expand your earning power? If you write your own nursing diagnosis for each obstacle encountered, you'll know what you have to do.

5. Get your questions answered before making any decisions. Don't talk yourself out of what you want. Get all the facts first….then make an informed decision.

6. Take small steps toward your goal. Take one class instead of three. Start small for big results.

Fall: Nurses! The Benefits of Making Mistakes

This month, I want to share with you the benefits of making mistakes. Many times, as health care professionals, we have every intention of doing a great job for everyone but ourselves. We read the best books to learn everything we can about what we do, and in the process we learn what study habits are most successful.

Eventually, in the medical field, we fall. We make a mistake and forget something relevant or significant. *How do you handle your mistakes? Are you your own worst critic, or do you have hecklers? Did you accidentally forget to unclamp your secondary tubing for your IV antibiotic?*

Making a mistake provides us with a new perspective and a set of information from a completely different vantage point. It is only when we fall that we come to know what the other possibilities are. Many times we continue to do things in the same old way, and we never have the benefit of seeing different outcomes. We can use our mistakes as learning opportunities to either get more information, to change unnecessary pressure from fix routines, or simply to laugh.

Secondly, everyone makes mistakes. Erase your need for perfection and replace it with understanding. Understand that you are human, and that you are doing your best as a nurse. Maybe you did put a wet-to-dry dressing on backward. This is insignificant in the big context of life. Maybe you missed the school play because you signed up to work overtime and it simply slipped your mind. This provides you with any opportunity to discuss how nurses—like everyone—make errors, and when they do, they have to be honest and courageous about what happened.

Thirdly, surround yourself with people who affirm and support you as you grow in this stage of your life. Sometimes we feel the need to show others that we are really good at this life as individuals. *Remember, that you have to do your best... not impress.* Nurses often ask me simple strategies to address others who question their individuality. I recommend the following steps to relieve this stress:

1. Establish some boundaries. Remember, we teach others how to treat us by what we allow.

2. Ask clearly but politely that physicians, coworkers, parents and friends who criticize and complain about your professional style or approach give you some space. You might say, "What you said to me hurt my feelings just now. I am learning and doing my best. You have to give me some room here."

3. Trust yourself. Know that your best is good enough. They don't make capes with a big gold "N" on the back. It's okay not to be Super-Nurse.

Remember, that no one is perfect and that you don't need to be perfect to be a terrific professional and individual. Being a good nurse requires love, commitment and nurturing. If your style contains any combination of those adjectives then your **mistakes** are **minor** and your **care** is **major**.

Great Self-Care Equals Great Health-Care

How is your health? What do you do to stay fit on the inside as well as the outside? When did you last visit the doctor?

What about you? How is your health? Are you able to share your health story? Is your health picture one of success or neglect? As health care professionals we have a responsibility to care for ourselves. We deserve to be healthy. Great health is a choice. We have the opportunity to choose every day to set the alarm one hour earlier in order to go on a walk. We can choose whether fast food is part of our daily health regime.

Some of the major causes of death, including heart disease, cancer, stroke, lung disease and injury, can be prevented through diet, weight loss and exercise. While we cannot prevent all things that happen to us physically, we can slow down the aging process by fueling our body with the diet and exercise it needs to thrive.

As you think about your health, consider your patients. Your patients are watching you. They are watching the example we set, whether it is a healthy example or one of neglect. What are they learning from you? What we do speaks so much more loudly than what we say. Are you setting an example? "Don't do as I do – do as I say", should never leave your lips.

This month, make a commitment with me to apply some simple strategies to getting your health on track.

They are:

Schedule medical appointments with all of your doctors immediately. This includes your primary physician or any relevant specialist. Make your health picture crystal clear.

Establish a consistent exercise routine. Take a walk with the family after dinner. Rake the leaves with your children on the weekends and play. Make exercise fun! Start a walking club with nurses from the unit. If it is too cold to go outside, consider exercises that you can do indoors, like the stairs at the hospital. Many hospitals now have a gym for tenured staff to use.

Eat Healthy. Purchase snacks that are low in sodium and processed sugars. Instead, snack on healthy foods, like broccoli, carrots or apple slices. Preparing healthy meals together is a terrific way to create quality time while educating on food choices. Create fun ways to eat foods that are high in fiber, fresh fruits and vegetables. Do it with the nurses you work with!

Decrease toxic activities, like drinking and smoking. It is a fact that one out of six deaths in the United States is blamed on smoking. Listen to your body, and minimize the harmful effects of tobacco and alcohol. Reduce others exposure to second-hand smoke.

Lose weight. Make time to play. Find ways to make yourself move in ways you enjoy. Park the car a few blocks away from work and walk.

Re-discover old hobbies. A hobby is a terrific way to become fit by doing something that you love. Join a softball league, yoga class, or swim team. Create healthy outlets to increase your health.

Being healthy is a necessity, not a luxury. Respecting your body and giving it what it requires will aid you in the long run. Change those bad habits into healthy choices.

Caring for yourself means caring about your quality of life. Remember that self-care is not negotiable, but necessary to being the best individual possible.

Nurses! Don't Let Your Life Schedule You.

Do you define self-love as a selfish act that results in diminished care and concern for the others in your life? When was the last time you treated yourself lovingly? What did you do for yourself?

Don't let your life schedule you.

Does the beginning of a new job have you stressed out? Have you found that since the start of a new shift you lack energy?

You are not alone. For most people, the routine unfolds slowly. Although most of us have a plan of how our schedule should run the best way to reduce stress and anxiety is to establish a new routine as soon as possible. In addition, everyone always performs better when they know what to expect.

In my case, my family enjoys summertime because it allows them the opportunity to sleep in and get extra rest. In order to get adjusted to the new routine, I rearrange bedtimes to reflect the children's school schedule three weeks before school begins. When school starts I recommend the following strategies for getting a family routine scheduled as soon as possible:

• Establish a set bed time routine and stick to it. We all perform better when rested. The American Academy of Pediatrics' Guide to Your Child's Sleep provides some helpful guidelines regarding how much sleep children need at different developmental stages. These numbers represent the recommended total number of hours of sleep in a 24-hour period. So, remember to add those naps into your numbers. They recommend the following:

AGE	HOURS OF SLEEP NEEDED
Birth-Six Months	16-20
Six-Twelve Months	14-15
1-3 Years	10-13
3-10 Years	10-12
11-12 Years	~10
Teenagers	~9
Adults	8-9
Elderly	5-9

• Do you have children? Have them pack their book bags the night before. Make sure that the notebooks and all other school supplies are in the backpack to avoid frustration and the mad morning search. These unexpected events usually contribute to their being late for school and their parents for and work. Teach children to check their book bags before they go to bed to make sure they have what they need. For younger children, create a check list of what their book bag needs so they can check it off each day.

• Are you tired of making meals that no one eats? Take a family survey on the best breakfast meals that everyone agrees on - to eat each week. This prevents you from creating delicious meals that go to waste. Ask family members to collectively decide on five different meals for breakfast. Tell them that if they eat the food that they suggest then they can help plan the breakfast menu for the following week.

• Teach your family how to pack their own lunches. Everyone loves taking ownership of their lunches. It is a wonderful way to increase the chances that lunch will be consumed instead of trashed, especially with children.

• Prepare your dinner in advance. Bulk cook on the weekends and freeze dinner for each day of the week. This will give you more time to Nurture-Me.

• Put a family calendar on the fridge that allows you to list all upcoming Events, meetings, and outings.. Having a calendar will ensure that family members know what is going on and when, so no important dates are missed.

• Minimize extra-curricular activities. This is tough to do at first, but helps reduce anxiety and stress. It is difficult for a nurse to leave work, run errands, play taxi, run to the store…all while the stress of the day if fresh on your mind.

• Commit some family time to having dinner together each week. Teach your children the importance of quiet and reflective time together as a family. Create a time after dinner to share important highlights about each day.

• Minimize stress by being proactive and creating a plan. Taking the time to schedule your life will prevent your life from scheduling you. Remember that self-care is not negotiable, but is necessary to be the best person possible.

Nurses! Exercise Choice In Your Life.

Are your self-care muscles weak? Do you suffer from indecision, complacency or the whatever-you-want syndrome? Do you pass up opportunities for yourself because you are afraid to simply commit.

Let's talk about the benefits of choice.

I love coaching nurses! Specifically, I love helping health care professionals realize their dreams, plans and goals. As a coach, I have found that most health care professionals are challenged with giving themselves the green light to live their lives. **Is this you?**

Perhaps you have a group of neighbors who walk together in the morning who want you participate. Or, maybe you want to take an evening pottery class for your enjoyment. **What's stopping you?**

Most nurses create a list of reasons why they should not choose to do the things that add value to their lives. As nurses, we can easily create a list of more important things to accomplish.

I want to encourage you to put yourself at the top of the list. Your family and friends wants you to be happy, healthy and fulfilled!

This month, e-mail me your commitment story. Feel free to write one sentence or more. I want to know what your plans are for you.

Here are my four tips (using the acronym for **L.I.S.T.**) for exercising choice in your life.

L List 10 things that you want to accomplish (e.g., exercise, make a new friend, or pursue a hobby or passion).

I Investigate your options. Many times we fail to pursue the things we love because we do not have enough information.. Get in touch with an old friend to schedule lunch at the hospital. Get your questions answered.

S Stop making excuses and start making connections. Ask yourself, "How can this work?" Look for the possibilities to create the opportunities that you want.

T Take time to live your dreams daily! Pursue your passion.

S.U.M.M.E.R.

Nurses, are you ready for the summer? What plans have you made for your family? This is designed to give you some ideas of how to make this the best summer ever for your family.

Here are my seven strategies for making the most of **S.U.M.M.E.R.** They are as follows:

Send out invitations to arrange social get-togethers with family and friends. The summer provides terrific opportunities to catch up with long lost friends or family members. Take some time to create a list of people you want to see this summer. Invite them over for a cookout, a visit to the pool, or coordinate a joint family vacation.

Uncover easy and simple things to do at home with your family. Blow off the dust from your family board games and play them instead of storing them. Remember the sprinkler in the backyard? Turn on the sprinkler for the children and take out umbrellas to use as shields. Look for easy ways to have fun at home. *No gas or cash necessary.*

Move every day. Take a walk through your neighborhood or visit a local park/playground. The American Heart Foundation recommends that we take a minimum of 10,000 steps a day. Look for easy ways to move together as a family.. Write down five ways to move together as a family. Encourage family fitness while having fun.

Make reading a part of every day. Visit the local library and select three favorite books to read over a two-week period. Every day give yourself time to read. Children who become fluent and strong readers usually do so as a result of others' commitment to read to them. (Nurses, while your children are reading, read for yourself.)

Eat well. The summer is a terrific time to modify diets to include all of the wonderful summer fruits and vegetables. Set a goal to eat a minimum of one fruit or vegetable at every meal. For example, at breakfast you might prepare a fruit salad with pineapple, strawberries, honeydew and blueberries with granola. At lunch you could serve raw broccoli, celery and carrot sticks with a light sandwich. With dinner, you could make spinach, walnut and apple salad along with some grilled kebobs. It is really that simple.

Reorganize your home. Clean out those closets and purge the unnecessary. When de-cluttering, create bins for things to keep, things to donate and things to get rid of. Do you have a collection of things that are unused? Give Help reduce clutter in your living environment.

My strategies for **S.U.M.M.E.R.** will aid you in having a meaningful, productive and healthy summer for all. Enjoy!

Self-Care for Nurses who are Parents

The demands of family life are exhausting. Carpooling, school activities, and birthday parties are just some of the many things we support in our children's lives. As parents, it is easy to become so inundated taking care of our children that we forget to nurture ourselves. This month, let's make a commitment to nurture ourselves. Our children are counting on us to set the right examples for them to follow. Let's teach them the value of self-care. By doing so, we illustrate to our children the importance of loving ourselves and what we do.

When we take time to care for ourselves, we feel empowered and are better able to accomplish more in our lives. Caring for ourselves permits us to love everyone around us better. As a result, we become more giving, grateful, and happy. By establishing quality adult time, we can connect and reflect on who we really are and what we really want. When did you last time consider what was best for you? When was the last time you relaxed in your favorite chair and enjoyed a cup of coffee? How many minutes each day do you get to connect with your spouse? Making the commitment to improve the quality of each day is a decision. Take small steps to enhance your life.

As the mother of three children between one and eight years old, I know first-hand the challenges that parents face. My husband and I make time every month to consistently nurture ourselves and our relationship. I believe that the best parents are ones that place their self-care as a priority. The benefits to our children are immediate when we take better care of ourselves. By sowing self-care into our lives we reap the benefits of reduced personal stress, anxiety and frustration.

Follow my five strategies for renewing the Self:

Rest
Find time to be still every day. Take the time to stop the roller coaster of life and slow down. When we are rested, we make better decisions. Better decisions equals less stress.

Read
Renew your mind. Fall in love with reading again. In my home, we Drop Everything And Read (D.E.A.R). Set clear

expectations with your children that everyone is going to read individually for 15 minutes, thereby limiting interruptions. No excuses. Reading allows us to escape the pressures of the day and allows us to expand our minds.

Rejuvenate
Rejuvenate your spirit. Take some time each day to connect with your higher power. Pray, reflect and meditate to connect with your spirit and allow peace to work in your life.

Readjust
Readjust your priorities. Is your family too busy? This is a great question to ask. Is your family racing from Monday morning to Sunday evening? Limit your children's activities. Be realistic about each commitment. Are your family members trying to keep up with you?

Reward
Reward yourself. Go on a date with yourself, your spouse or a friend. Take some time away from the family and enjoy some grown-up time. When you return you will feel like a new person.

Making the decision to care for you is a deliberate choice. Choose to make self-care a priority. Remember that self-care is not negotiable, but necessary in order to be the best parent possible.

Don't forget to sign up for my free newsletter at www. findingdefinitions.com/caregivers.html

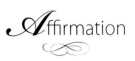

I took an action for me today and it felt great!

_____

(Your Signature)

_____

_____

_____

_____

_____

_____

_____

_____

_____

_____

_____

_____

_____

_____

_____

_____

_____

_____

$\mathcal{I}$n Conclusion…
The Next Steps

Now that you have read our book, we would like you use this section to record some of your personal goals, insights, solutions or favorite tips. Let's call this your "cheat sheet" to ensure that you remember what works best for you.

Review each chapter and record a personal discovery that you made regarding each chapter's strategy.

For each chapter ask yourself:

- What shift can I make today in this area of my life?

- What is my next step with my own self-care?

- What routines or rituals work best to keep me on a successful path?

- What are my self-care goals?

- Why are these goals important to me?

- How would my life be more fulfilling if I address this area of my life?

- How would my family benefit?

- What are the steps I must take to ensure my own self-care?

- What is the timeline for this goal?

- How can I use the DIPP strategy?

- How can I break this goal into smaller pieces?

Please remember to join us at www.findingdefinitions.com/caregivers.html and join other health care professionals just like you who are Finding Time to Care for Me.

Thank you for committing to your own success.

Live Fully,
Mia and Lorna

_____
_____
_____
_____
_____
_____
_____
_____
_____
_____
_____
_____
_____
_____
_____
_____
_____
_____
_____
_____
_____
_____
_____
_____
_____
_____
_____

_____

_____

_____

_____

_____

_____

_____

_____

_____

_____

_____

_____

_____

_____

_____

_____

_____

_____

_____

_____

_____

_____

_____

_____

_____

_____

Journal Pages

Breinigsville, PA USA
08 September 2009
223611BV00005B/4/P